This guide is a must-have for all medical school applicants! With her insider's view, Jennifer Welch offers realistic advice that makes the dreaded application process more clear, and honest tips to helping candidates avoid often fatal flaws. I wish I had had this when I applied to medical school!

Jason L. Freedman, M.D.
Pediatrics Resident
Columbia University Medical Center

This book provides a comprehensive and practical guide on how to navigate successfully the medical school application process. In addition to clarifying the many tangible requirements that are necessary to be competitive, Jennifer Welch gives the reader a window into the intangibles that significantly impact an admissions decision. An excellent read for both the savvy and the "clueless" medical school applicant.

Paula Jacobs
Senior Associate Director
Student and Career Development
College of Human Ecology
Cornell University

101 Tips on Getting into Medical School

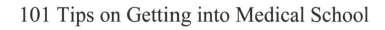

101 TIPS
—— on getting into ——
MEDICAL
SCHOOL

Jennifer C. Welch

>> North Syracuse, New York <<
<< Gegensatz Press >>
>> 2007 <<

Cataloging-in-Publication:

Welch, Jennifer C. (Jennifer Cox), 1971-
  101 tips on getting into medical school / Jennifer C. Welch.
    128 p. ; 22 cm.
    "Jennifer C. Welch, M.S., is the Director of Admissions at the
sixteenth oldest medical school in the United States."
    ISBN 978-1-933237-06-0
1. Medical colleges—United States—Admissions. 2. Medical colleges—United
States—Entrance requirements. 3. Premedical education—United States.
[DNLM: 1. Schools, Medical. 2. School Admission Criteria. 3. United States.
W 19 W439o 2007]
I. Title. II Title: One hundred and one tips on getting into medical school.
    R838.4 W44o 2007   610.71/173—dc22   AACR2
Library of Congress Control Number 2006936128

First edition, first printing. Printed in the United States of America by United
Book Press, Baltimore, Maryland..

The guillemets, or two pairs of opposing chevrons, dark on the lower cusps and
light on the upper, are a trademark of Gegensatz Press.

Distributed to the trade worldwide by:
Gegensatz Press
108 Deborah Lane
North Syracuse, NY 13212-1931
<www.gegensatzpress.com>

Cover design by Sabra Snyder.
Cover photograph by Deborah Rexine.
Interior design by Eric v.d. Luft.
Printed on acid-free paper. ∞

Contents

The Interview Process 73

About the Author

Jennifer Welch has worked in college admissions since 1993 and has advised thousands of students in preparing their applications to college. As a school counselor and a college admissions professional, she has been a successful liaison between prospective students and various academic institutions on both the secondary and collegiate level.

Since 2001 she has served as Director of Admissions at the State University of New York (SUNY) Upstate Medical University, one of North America's oldest medical schools. In this capacity, she has guided thousands of prospective students through the entire application process, evaluated thousands of student applications, participated as a voting member on several admissions committees, visited hundreds of colleges and universities, and has developed successful recruitment strategies. In 2006 she founded CollegeBound101 <www.collegebound101.com>, an educational consulting company dedicated to helping students maneuver through the college admissions process.

She received a bachelor of arts degree in economics from the SUNY College at Potsdam and a master of science degree in school counseling from Syracuse University. She lives in Marcellus, New York, with her husband, Dennis, and their three children.

Preface

This book is designed to provide applicants with an "inside" perspective on the medical school application and admission process. Too often applicants delay their applications or hurt their chances of admission by heeding the wrong advice, or making assumptions about what is required or acceptable in the application process.

Prospective students should use this as a guide in preparing for the often overwhelming process of applying to medical school. The book attempts to clarify that process and help students avoid some common mistakes. It is intended to provide real-world practical advice about how to navigate the complex medical college admissions process. While there are Web sites, books, and physicians that may be able to provide applicants with information and advice regarding the admissions process, few of these sources are actually able to speak from the inside point of view of an admissions director. These tips are based on years of experience from someone who has actively helped to set the standards for, and played an integral role in, selecting the incoming classes for a medical school.

The information provided in this book is by no means a guarantee of acceptance. For concrete information about each medical school, applicants should check directly with the admissions office at that school. Contact information on each medical school is listed in the back of this book.

Acknowledgments

This book would not have been possible without the knowledge, encouragement, mentoring, friendship, and vision of Dr. E. Gregory Keating, Dean of Student Affairs and Associate Dean of Admissions at SUNY Upstate Medical University, 2001-2006. We were looking forward to writing this book together until Greg's very untimely and tragic death in August 2006. No one was more dedicated to students and their success than Greg. Not a day goes by that I do not think about him and miss his humor, support, drive, positive attitude, his passion for life, and his work.

I am so thankful to my family for all of their love and support while putting this book together. To my husband, thank you for listening to me and for your support. To my children, I love you to the moon and back — you are my inspiration and my life. To my parents, sisters, and sister-in-law, whose love, support, and encouragement got me here, thank you for everything. To my two best friends, who would have thought?

A very special thank you to Isabelle Rhoades, my close friend and colleague, for keeping me focused while writing this book. I am so appreciative for your feedback, ideas, editing assistance and comic relief. I could not have done this without you!

Thank you to Debbie Rexine for a great photo and Sabra Snyder for a fabulous cover design. You are both truly talented.

Thank you to Candace Rhea, Sally Sutphen, and Linda Linn for all of your editing assistance and for all of the help in making this book flow. I really appreciate all of your efforts.

To Eric Luft, Ph.D., thank you for making this book come to life! I am not sure I would have gotten this far without you! Greg would be proud that we were able to do this together.

To Carolyn Couch and Carol Morath, thank you both so much for taking such good care of me all of these years. You make my job and life so much easier. Thank you to Donna Vavonese, Joni Hinds, Leah Caldwell, and Susan Stearns, Ph.D., for all of your ideas, encouragement, honesty, and assistance!

To Lynn Cleary, M.D., Senior Associate Dean of Education and current Dean of Student Affairs, thank you for giving me the opportunity to put this book together and for the encouragement and feedback you have provided along the way.

Thank you to Joni Huff, Director of Admissions, Pritzker School of Medicine at the University of Chicago and previous pre-health advisor at Yale University; Paula Jacobs, pre-health advisor at Cornell University; and Eileen Sharp, pre-health advisor at Wilkes University, for taking the time to read the manuscript and provide me with such valuable feedback. It is great to have such wonderful colleagues who are as dedicated to students and as passionate as you are about seeing students succeed in the health professions.

To Scott Cameron, Ph.D., MSII, Nikki Gero, M.B.A., MSIII (a.k.a. the eternal medical student), Cameron Hall, MSII, Rajitha Devadoss, MSII, Joshua Nelson, MSI, TeSha English, MSI, and Jason Freedman, M.D., PGY2 Columbia University — thank you so much for taking the time out of your incredibly busy schedules to help me with this book. I know you will all be fabulous physicians.

Two authoritative Web sites furnished me with extensive and substantial data: the AAMC page on "Facts — Applicants, Matriculants and Graduates" <www.aamc.org/data/facts/2006/2006mcatgpa.htm>, used on page 42; and the E-Zine at CollegeGrad.com. "The Most Important Interview Non-Verbals." <www.collegegrad.com/ezine/21nonver.shtml>, quoted on pages 96 and 97.

This book is dedicated to the memory of E. Gregory Keating, Ph.D. I could not have asked for a better mentor, supervisor, or friend.

Getting Ready

The following information is for prospective medical students to use as a general guideline in the application and admissions process for medical school. Each undergraduate college may do things a little differently, so it is important for you to reach out to the resources that are available to you on your campus. Your pre-health advisor will play a key role in helping you prepare for this huge undertaking. Make sure you work closely with him/her.

1 Be aware of all of the reasons why you are interested in a medical career.

You must be confident that a medical career is something you are deeply committed to, and you must be able to convey that commitment both verbally and in writing. Simply saying that you have always wanted to be a physician because you want to "help people" or that you enjoy watching *House* or *ER* will not be enough. Spend some time really thinking about all of the reasons why you are doing this, and be sure that your reasons are thoughtful, clear, and true to the person you are.

If you are convinced that medical school is the right path for you, be sure that you are doing it for all of the "right" reasons, and know what you are getting yourself into. You will eventually need to convince medical school admissions committees that you are genuinely motivated to pursue a career in medicine. Be sure you can answer the "Why medicine?" question. There are many careers which "help people." Why have you chosen medicine instead of deciding to be a physician assistant, nurse, physical therapist, medical radiographer, social worker, or biology teacher?

Getting into medical school is not easy. Less than half of the students who apply to medical school each year will be accepted. Medical schools are looking for the most intelligent and motivated students they can find. Successful applicants will need to demonstrate a clear desire to work with and help people, will need to work hard, and will need to be committed to the field of medicine.

2 Be realistic about your chances for admission.

A 2.0 cumulative grade point average (GPA) and a single-digit combined Medical College Admissions Test (MCAT) score will not get you into medical school. Take the time to research thoroughly the schools you plan on applying to and be realistic about your chances of gaining admission to medical school. Research your target medical schools' average MCAT test scores and GPAs. Many schools have this information available on their Web sites, and contact information for each medical school is listed at the end of this book.

**Medical College Admission Test
(MCAT)**
www.aamc.org/mcat

The MCAT Care Team
Association of American Medical Colleges
Section for Applicant Assessment Services
2450 N Street, NW
Washington, DC 20037
Phone: (202) 828-0690

Most U.S. medical schools require applicants to
submit MCAT scores. The MCAT is broken down
into four different categories: Verbal Reasoning,
Physical Sciences, Writing Sample, and Biological
Sciences. The highest score you can obtain in each
of the Verbal Reasoning, Physical Science, and
Biological Science areas is 15. The Writing Sample
is scored using an alpha system, with the lowest
score of "J" and the highest of "T".

Purchase the current edition of the *Medical School
Admissions Requirements* (*MSAR*) book that is put
together each year by the Association of American
Medical Colleges (AAMC). GPA and MCAT averages
may change from year to year. Your pre-health advisor
may also have a copy of this book for you to use as a
reference.

**Association of American Medical Colleges
(AAMC)**
www.aamc.org/students

The AAMC is a very useful reference tool as you
begin the medical school application process. The
web site contains information on each medical
school, contact information, various publications,
student responsibility information, medical school
responsibility information, tips on applying to
medical school, financial planning information,
information for minority students, and health
professions advisor information.

3 Visit with your pre-med advisor often and early.

If you are currently in college, it is very important to
maintain close contact with your pre-health or pre-med
advisor. A mistake that many students make in this process
is either not meeting with him/her at all, or meeting with
him/her too late. Your pre-health advisor is an invaluable
resource and should be sought out early in your college
career. He/she will be very helpful in assisting you through
this rather daunting experience. Be sure that you have a
good working relationship with your advisor and be sure to
take his/her advice seriously. In many cases, your advisor
will be the person responsible for providing your letter(s)

of recommendation to medical schools. If you have a solid relationship with your advisor, he/she can provide a letter from someone who knows you well and can comment on your character, ambition, and suitability for a career in medicine. This more personal letter will be more effective than one simply stating that the writer has had one appointment with you, you arrived on time, and were pleasant and attentive during your meeting.

If there is no pre-health advisor on your campus or if you are a non-traditional student, the National Association of Advisors for the Health Professionals (NAAHP) advisor-at-large service may be able to provide you with some advice on applying to medical school. Its Web site <www.naahp.org> provides a list of members willing to volunteer their time to help applicants who do not have access to an advisor. There is also a list of colleges and universities that do have health professions advisors on campus.

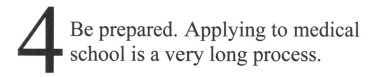 Be prepared. Applying to medical school is a very long process.

You must begin the application process more than a year in advance of when you hope to matriculate. A general timeline for traditional applicants might look something like this:

Freshman Year
Meet your pre-health advisor.
Get involved in the student run pre-health (or pre-med) groups.

Get off to a good start academically.
Begin extracurricular activities.
Look into opportunities for a medically related summer
  job or volunteer experience.

Summer Courses

It is best for students to complete medical school
prerequisites during the academic year at the
undergraduate college or university where they are
enrolled. If you must take summer courses to
complete your degree or complete another major, be
sure you do so at a similar type of college as the one
where you are matriculated. It is probably not in your
best interest to take courses at a two-year college.

Sophomore Year

Maintain contact with your pre-health advisor.
Attend any medically-related pre-health events and/or
  activities on your campus.
Maintain a solid academic record, by doing well and
  taking academically challenging courses each semester.
Continue your extracurricular involvement.
Get involved in research opportunities, if they interest
  you.
Look into opportunities for a medically related summer
  job or volunteer experience.

Look into participating in a summer medical careers program.
Begin looking into the different medical schools. This is a good time to purchase a copy of the *MSAR*.

Medical School Admissions Requirements (MSAR) Book

This is a "must-have" book. It has invaluable information on each participating medical school, including:

➤ Deadlines and requirements.
➤ The average GPAs and MCAT scores of matriculated students.
➤ Contact information for each medical school.
➤ Financial aid information, including tuition costs and special program information.

Purchase a copy of this book at <www.aamc.org/publications>, or ask your pre-health advisor if you can borrow a copy.

Junior Year
Continue to maintain a strong academic record.
Complete all medical school prerequisite requirements.
Continue your extracurricular involvement.
Meet with your pre-health advisor regularly.

Select your recommenders.
Interview with the pre-health committee.
Prepare for the MCATs.
Take the MCAT exam in the spring or early summer.
Familiarize yourself with the different application
    services: the American Medical College Application
    Service (AMCAS), the Texas Medical and Dental
    Schools Application Service (TMDSAS), and the
    American Association of Colleges of Osteopathic
    Medicine Application Service (AACOMAS).

American Medical College
Application Service
(AMCAS)
www.aamc.org/amcas

2450 N Street, NW
Washington, DC 20037-1123
E-mail: amcas@aamc.org
Phone: (202) 828-0600

AMCAS is a centralized processing center for first-year
applicants at participating Allopathic Medical Schools
in the United States. Please see the end of this book for
those schools currently participating in AMCAS.

Summer Between Junior and Senior Year
    Complete a medically related summer job or volunteer
    experience.

Participate in a summer medical careers program.
Narrow down the list of medical schools that you will be applying to.
Complete the application process through American Medical College Application Service (AMCAS).
Submit your application and all of your college transcripts to AMCAS.
Let your pre-health office know which schools you are applying to and where your letters of recommendation should be sent.
Request that your letters of recommendation be sent to your pre-health office.
Take the MCATs, if you have not already.
Complete any secondary applications you receive.

Texas Medical and Dental Schools
Application Service
(TMDSAS)
www.utsystem.edu/tmdsas/

702 Colorado, Suite 6.400
Austin, TX 78701
Phone (512) 499-4785

TMDSAS is a centralized processing center for students applying to the six allopathic medical schools in Texas. Please see the end of this book for the schools currently participating in TMDSAS.

Fall of Senior Year

Finish any outstanding secondary applications.
Make sure that your applications are complete at each of
the medical schools.
Interview at medical schools.
Continue to maintain a strong academic record.
Continue your extracurricular involvement.

**American Association of Colleges of Osteopathic
Medicine Application Service
(AACOMAS)**
aacomas.aacom.org/

5550 Friendship Boulevard
Suite 310
Chevy Chase, MD 20815-7231
Phone: (301) 968-4190
E-mail: aacomas@aacom.org

AACOMAS is the centralized processing center for
students applying to the twenty-six osteopathic
(DO) medical schools in the United States. There
are twenty-three colleges of osteopathic medicine
and three branch campuses.

Spring of Senior Year

Continue to maintain a strong academic record.
Begin looking into financial resources.

28

Submit the Free Application for Federal Student Aid
form (FAFSA) <www.fafsa.ed.gov>.
Attend Second Visit Days to help narrow down your
choices.
Finish the degree program you are enrolled in.
Make your final decision on which medical school you
will attend, and withdraw from the others no later than
May 15.

Multiple Acceptance Day
May 15

If you are fortunate enough to be accepted at multiple
schools, it is important to release multiple acceptances
as soon as you know where you will be attending
medical school. There is no reason for students to be
holding on to seven or eight acceptances at any given
time. There are so many other qualified applicants
waiting for openings at the various medical schools.
After May 15, medical schools may rescind an
acceptance to applicants that are holding more than
one medical school acceptance.

Summer after Senior Year

Send final transcripts to the medical school you will be
attending.
Attend orientation program.
Begin medical school!

5 Be prepared for the fact that applying to medical school can be a very expensive process.

During a one-year application cycle, you could spend $3,500-$5,000 just to apply to medical school:

> ➢ Initial AMCAS application fees.
> ➢ AMCAS application fee for each medical school you apply to. (Students typically apply to between fifteen and twenty medical schools.)
> ➢ Secondary application fees ($45-$100 a piece).
> ➢ Travel expenses (airfare, bus or train, taxis, parking).
> ➢ Hotel costs (one or two nights depending on distance and length of interview day).
> ➢ Interview clothes.
> ➢ Food.
> ➢ Other incidentals.

6 Dare to be different. Stand out in the application process!

There are far too many "cookie cutter" applicants who all look the same on paper and in black interview suits. You need to set yourself apart from all of the other applicants.

Figure out what is special about you and what you have to offer the field of medicine that is different from all of the other applicants. Get involved in a variety of activities and when you find something that you love, stick with it.

Participate in activities because you really want to do them and enjoy them, not because they will look good on your resume.

7 Major in whatever you want.

While it is true that the majority of applicants to medical school are or were science majors, you do not **have** to major in biology or chemistry. There are many other fascinating fields of study available: psychology, theatre arts, history, computer science, English, etc. If there is a particular program that you really want to pursue, do it!

Other majors will provide you with a different perspective on the field of medicine and could be looked upon very favorably by an admissions committee. Be careful about trying to impress medical schools by choosing programs of study that are viewed as more "difficult," such as neuroscience or biophysics. If the result is a much lower GPA, the admissions committee may doubt your ability to be successful in the basic science years of your medical school education.

8 Find a balance in your life.

You will need to juggle your academics, personal life, extracurricular activities, family, and personal time. Study hard, get involved, investigate the field of medicine, and love what you do.

Many people entering a health profession are combining their vocation and their avocation; they make their work their play. You will truly need to love this job. There will be many long and difficult days, and you must be passionate about what you are getting in to. Having a good balance of work and play will help you find release from the stress that you may end up facing on a daily basis.

9 Let the admissions office know if you are applying during the same application year as your husband, wife, or significant other.

Most medical schools are willing to cluster your interview schedules making it easier for you and the school.

10 Consider taking some time off between college and medical school.

Taking time off from academics before entering medical school is becoming more common, and it occurs for a variety of reasons: research opportunities, clinical experiences, traveling abroad, and family and/or financial reasons, such as working to pay off undergraduate student loans. It also may be a good time to decide if the medical profession is the right career for you. Medical schools are seeing more and more non-traditional applicants, including students who have been out of school for a while and may be changing careers. Many of these applicants wanted to be physicians earlier in their lives, but felt it was unattainable. Only now are they realizing that they should have followed their hearts from the beginning.

Medical schools want you to apply when you are ready. For some applicants that is right out of college and for others it is after years of pursuing another career, taking time to reflect, or starting a family. Be prepared to articulate clearly why you took time off or why you decided to change careers.

Applying To Medical School

The application that you submit to medical schools must be perfect! Spend a great deal of time putting it together. Everything that you submit in the application will be looked at and evaluated. Spell things correctly, use proper grammar, and appropriate punctuation. Keep in mind that there will be many people reviewing your application. Members of the admissions committee may have very different backgrounds and/or perspectives about potential medical school students, and they may not all be looking for the same things in your application.

It is also important not to think of applying to medical school as simply a checklist. ("If I do this, this, and this, then I will be accepted into medical school.") Every applicant is looked at as an individual and the admissions committee is hoping to find something different in each and every applicant. They often ask, "What can this student contribute to the field of medicine that is different from everyone else?"

With extracurricular activities, quality matters more than quantity. Choose activities that are meaningful to you. Your activities should reflect your personal and academic interests, and allow you to demonstrate qualities such as initiative, ability to handle responsibility, leadership skills, critical thinking skills, and a commitment to service work in your community.

What Medical Schools Look For In an Applicant

❖ Academic achievement.
❖ Meaningful experiences dealing with and relating to people.
  ➤ Extracurricular activities.
  ➤ Service volunteer work.
  ➤ Clinical experience.
❖ Character.
❖ Drive and motivation for a career in medicine.
  ➤ Personal statement.
  ➤ Interview — communication skills.

Thank you to E. Gregory Keating.

---

11 Apply early!

Medical school admission is very competitive so you must get your applications in **early**. Rolling admission does not mean that you can wait until the last possible minute to apply. Schools with rolling admission review applications as they come in. As students are accepted, there will be more competition for the smaller number of remaining spots available. Admissions committees now have a greater number of other applicants to compare with you for those few remaining seats. You are, in a sense, stacking the odds against yourself by procrastinating.

The AMCAS application process begins every year on May 1, and applicants may begin filling out their applications at that time. June 1 of each year is first day that applicants may submit their applications to AMCAS. It is not in your best interest to wait until right before a medical school's deadline to apply.

Here is the problem: if you apply to a medical school on November 1 (the AMCAS deadline for the medical school that you are applying to), you will meet that deadline, but if the medical school has a final deadline for a completed application of December 1, you may not make the medical school's own deadline. AMCAS is very clear that it may take four to six weeks to verify an application — and that is if everything goes smoothly. It is not uncommon for additional information to be requested, delaying the verification of your initial AMCAS application and, in turn, delaying your application from being received and/or reviewed by the medical schools of your choice. Clearly, it is not in an applicant's best interest to wait until the very last day to apply to medical school. You will not be able to meet the medical school's final deadline.

This is also true of schools that do not have rolling admission, such as Harvard, Yale, and Johns Hopkins. It is always in your best interest to apply early when more interview positions are available.

While deadline extensions can be requested, they are rarely granted. To avoid the complication of requesting an extension, start the application process early and be proactive. Keep in mind the kind of impression you are making on the admissions committee when you have to request additional time in order to complete your application. Enrolling in medical school and later becoming a physician requires a great deal of responsibility, organization, and time management. Your inability to meet a deadline for which you are allotted ample time might speak volumes about how you will perform in the future.

12 If you call the admissions office, always ask with whom you are speaking, write down their name, the date of your call, and the reason for your call.

If, for example, your application was late and you called to get an extension, you must be able to verify that deadline extension was granted by someone in the admissions office.

If you need permission to deviate from the stated policies, be sure you know to whom you are speaking and mark the date and time. Then follow-up with an e-mail confirming what you were told.

13 Include everything in your application that you really want the admissions committee to know about you.

It is important for the admissions committee to know ifyou have experience working with the elderly, volunteering at a boys' and girls' club, or shadowing a doctor while you were in high school. These experiences tell the committee that you have an interest in serving others. As a physician, you will be dedicating your life to serving other people, and it is important that you have evidence of this in your application. Even an experience such as waiting on tables shows that you have had experience managing your time, dealing with difficult people, and multitasking.

Include all clinically related or volunteer experiences in the activities section of your application instead of giving them a brief mention in your personal statement. If an admissions officer is scanning your application during an initial review, these relevant experiences may be very easily overlooked. List the experiences. Make them easily identifiable and very clear. Do not make an admissions person search for them. It could make a difference in the outcome of your application.

Elements of a Good Application

- ➢ Imagine the reader.
- ➢ Be perfect in grammar.
- ➢ Have no typos.
- ➢ Be succinct.
- ➢ Be understated.
- ➢ Be honest.

Thank you to E. Gregory Keating.

14

Do not leave it up to the admissions committee to decide why your grades were so poor during a particular semester.

If your grades were weak during a particular semester or year, it is important that you address this somewhere in your application or in a letter to the admissions committee.

Do not leave it to up to the admissions committee to determine what was going on in your life during that time. The committee will notice the inconsistency in your grades, and they will wonder if you are trying to hide something. Do not make excuses about what was going on. Just be honest and straightforward.

Admissions committees look for a progression of grades. They want to be sure that as you take more challenging courses each year, your GPA continues to rise.

15 Make sure you have a professional contact e-mail address.

E-mail addresses such as <drgoodluv@hotmail.com>, <imastud247@yahoo.com>, or <Qteepie@gmail.com> are inappropriate to use when applying to medical school. Addresses such as these can tell an admissions committee a lot about your character that you do not even realize.

16 If you have a page on Facebook, MySpace, or YouTube make sure it is professional.

Attending medical school is the first professional step in the process of becoming a physician. You need to act in a professional way from the beginning of the application process. Sites like Facebook, MySpace, or YouTube can be a great way to stay in touch with friends, but as with all things, you **never** want to put anything on these sites that could reflect a less-than-professional aspect of your personality. Admissions committees may not have time to look at these sites for every applicant, but it is a **very** small world out there. Be careful.

17

Do not inundate the admissions committee with supplemental materials such as CDs, videos, DVDs, portfolios, or full three-ring binders.

Admissions committee members do not have the time to read all of these supplemental materials. In most cases, you are welcome to send a brief update indicating an abstract, information on a recent publication, new clinical experiences, or something special that you have accomplished, but do not send volumes of new information. Chances are, it will not be reviewed.

18

Do not argue with or be rude to any member of the admissions office staff.

Be polite and pleasant to all your contacts in the admissions office. If you are rude or inconsiderate to the support or clerical staff, it may get back to the admissions director and/or the admissions committee, and it could have damaging effects on your candidacy for admission. Remember, how you present yourself says something about how, as a physician, you will interact with your patients, colleagues, office personnel, and subordinates.

19 Do not inundate the admissions office with repeated phone calls.

When you must call to ask a question, trust that the answer is correct. You are dealing with admissions professionals who follow their medical school policy and answer many of the same questions every day. If you have a concrete reason to be skeptical of the response you are getting from the staff, ask to speak to the director.

Use common sense. Calling the admissions office every day will probably work against you.

20 Be realistic about the number of schools you apply to.

It is appropriate to apply to fifteen to twenty medical schools, but select them carefully. Talk to your pre-health advisor and/or use the *MSAR* to see which schools are the best for you to apply to, based on location, grades, test scores, type of teaching, and any other factors that are important to you.

It is also important to consider applying to a wide range of schools. You might be surprised to be rejected from a school where your GPA and MCAT scores are higher than its average. On the other hand, one of your "reach" schools might see something unique about you or your application and accept you. A good mix might be to apply to state schools and private schools where your statistics are competitive, and also apply to one or two "reach" schools. Stay away from applying to schools outside your home state if they only accept two or three out-of-state applicants per year.

According to the AAMC, 39,108 people applied to medical school for the 2006 entering class. 17,370 (44.4%) accepted students ended up enrolling at one of the 125 U.S. allopathic medical schools.

Applicants and Matriculants to U.S.
Allopathic Medical Schools
AAMC Statistics on the 2006 Entering Class

Average overall GPA of applicants: 3.48
Average science GPA of applicants: 3.38
Average MCAT of applicants: 27.6 (O)

Average overall GPA of matriculants: 3.64
Average science GPA of matriculants: 3.57
Average MCAT of matriculants: 30.4 (P)

21 Take challenging courses.

Admissions committees take into consideration the courses you take and how you position them. Be sure to discuss this with your pre-health advisor. You want to take challenging courses, preferably two science courses, each with a lab, and other challenging coursework. Be sure to take full course loads each semester and be careful not to add a lot of "fluff" courses. Earning a 3.7 for a semester in which you carried a full course load including several upper-level science courses will almost always carry more weight than a 3.9 earned for a semester when you took one rigorous science course surrounded by "fluff" courses like jazzercise or introduction to origami. It is important really to challenge yourself and prove to the admissions committee that you can handle a rigorous academic course load.

22 Do not blame your professors for your poor grades.

Do not try to make excuses for, or try to defend, your poor grades. If you are invited for an interview be prepared to discuss those grades, but instead of placing the blame on someone else, focus on the positive and perhaps highlight your academic performance since then. Emphasize what you learned from the experience, such as adjusting your study habits, taking advantage of office hours, curtailing your extracurricular activities, and learning to manage your time better.

Even in medical school, you may have an instructor whose teaching style does not match your learning style, and you may need to learn the material on your own. Berating a professor or maligning his/her character will not win the admissions interviewer to your side. Not all professors are equally effective in the classroom and not all material is equally interesting to students. This is a reality in every academic setting.

You should present yourself as a person who is committed to achieving goals without blaming others when you encounter difficulties. This also speaks to how you will approach the heavy course load and different teaching styles within a medical institution.

23 Do not make excuses for poor MCAT scores.

Right after the MCAT scores are released, phones go wild in medical school admissions offices. It will not help to panic over disappointing scores, and blaming your scores on "bad sushi" the day of the exam will only make it worse. Take responsibility for your disappointing scores, and be honest with yourself and the medical schools you are applying to.

Re-taking the MCAT many times could have a negative impact on your application unless there is a dramatic change in the scores. Though there is no longer a rule against repeating the MCATs more than three times, doing so probably will not work in your favor.

Though some medical schools may average your test scores or take the highest score in each subtest, most consider your most recent test scores the most important in the application process.

Keep in mind that most schools will only accept MCAT scores that are less than three years old, and there are some medical schools that will only accept them if they are less than two years old.

24 Know how to overcome a low GPA and/or MCAT score.

GPA and MCAT scores are usually the first items that medical schools look to when evaluating a student's application. Grades and MCATs combined carry 65% to 70% of the weight in the admissions decision. Admissions committees want to be sure that, if you are accepted, you will be academically successful in medical school and ultimately be successful on your National Boards. The National Board exams are taken at the conclusion of the second and fourth years of medical school. MCATs play a bigger role in the admissions decision now that students are required to take shelf exams during their clerkship years. MCATs have proven to be a positive predictor of a student's ability to pass these exams.

Be sure you have completed all the medical school prerequisites prior to sitting for the MCAT. The MCATs are offered many different times over the course of the year, so do not feel pressure to take them until you are ready. In April of the junior year students are normally finishing either physics II or organic chemistry II, preparing for finals in all their other courses, getting ready to apply to medical school, and studying for the MCAT. Take your time and think about taking the May or June exams. This will give you the opportunity to finish your course work, take your final exams, and then have some time to study for the MCATs without feeling so much pressure to do it all at once.

If you know you have difficulty with standardized tests, or if you perform poorly the first time you take the MCATs, consider taking an MCAT prep course through Kaplan or the Princeton Review. Often, however, time and financial restraints prevent routine enrollment in MCAT prep courses.

If your MCAT scores are not what you had hoped, try to pinpoint your area of weak performance, but do not focus exclusively on that area as you prepare to take the exam again. You may need to bring your Verbal Reasoning scores up, but not at the expense of Biological Science or Physical Science. Try to stay balanced in preparing for the exam.

If your GPA, particularly your science GPA, is not as high as it should or could be to apply to medical school and your grades fluctuated greatly over the course of your college career, consider completing a master's degree in the hard sciences before applying to medical school. There are several one-year master's programs that you might want to consider. For instance, the programs at Boston University, Georgetown University, and Johns Hopkins University prepare students well for the medical school curriculum. These programs allow students to take medical school courses with current medical students and provide the students with very good medical school advising.

Other strong "record enhancing" programs in the Northeast are at Drexel University and Duquesne University. Any graduate program offering a master's degree in the sciences would be a possibility. Discuss your options with your pre-health advisor. There are also special programs designed for students underrepresented in medicine, such as Southern Illinois University's Medical/Dental Education Preparatory Program (MEDPREP).

If you came late to the decision to enter medical school or did not take the science prerequisites as an undergraduate, look for a post-baccalaureate program designed to give students interested in medicine the prerequisite courses they will need to apply to medical school. Check out the AAMC's post-baccalaureate premedical programs search engine at <services.aamc.org/postbac/> for information on various programs. There are programs available that focus on applicants making a career change, applicants that need to enhance their academic records, minority applicants, and economically or educationally disadvantaged applicants.

25 Do not apply to medical school just because your parents want you to.

This may seem obvious, but medical school has to be **your** dream. Do not apply to medical school because of cultural pressure or because your father/mother wanted to become a doctor but could not. Everyone understands familial pressure, but you have to really want this for you! If you are not completely open, honest, and passionate about pursuing a career in medicine, it is going to be a very long, hard road. If your disingenuous pursuit of medicine does not come through during your interview, it will come through within the first few years of medical school when your true interests will clash with the time and pressures of your medical school courses. Medical school is a tremendous gift to those who attend and comes at great expense in time and money. Likewise, every person who serves at the medical school is dedicated to see you succeed in your pursuit. Medical school personnel invest in you in every way possible: personal commitment, time, and financially. Do not take this leap if you have doubts.

26 Be very careful when expressing any real or perceived personal connections during the admissions process.

Saying things like "Do you know who my father/mother is?" may not have the effect you had hoped for. The process of applying to, being accepted, and ultimately going to medical school is an independent process. You need to present yourself as an independent entity with the ability to obtain admission without acting as the child of … Your ability to express yourself as an individual will make a more positive impression on those who are reviewing your record.

Eventually you will need to make quick decisions without relying on who you know or who you are related to. Chances are your father or mother is not going to be there when you have a life or death decision to make about one of your future patients.

27 Do not have your parents call to check on the status of your application.

By the time you apply to medical school, you really should be an independent student, doing things for yourself. Even if you do not think you have the time, make the time. It does not look good to an admissions committee when you cannot call on your own behalf to inquire about how your medical school application is progressing. For confidentiality reasons, the admissions staff will not release information about your application or discuss the status of your application with your parents and/or spouse at any time anyway. Having them call on your behalf reflects badly on you.

28 Check with each medical school about its requirements, because each medical school may have different prerequisites.

Check with each medical school or take a look at the *MSAR*

to see what courses each school will require for admission. Some will require the basic pre-medical courses:

General biology I and II with a lab
General chemistry I and II with a lab
General physics I and II with a lab (some may require calculus-based physics)
Organic chemistry I and II with a lab
English courses

Other medical schools may require calculus, statistics, biochemistry, humanities, and/or social science courses.

Take some additional courses that may be helpful for you during your basic science years. These include physiology, cell/molecular biology, histology, biochemistry, and genetics. They will be helpful in providing you with a solid foundation when completing your first two years of medical school.

Course work in the humanities, public health, the social sciences, expository writing, and ethics are also encouraged. Physicians must have strong interpersonal and communication skills and must be able to express their thoughts and ideas clearly. They also must have strong decision-making skills, be able to think independently, and be able to read and understand scientific writings.

Some medical schools do not have specific prerequisites, but recommend many of the above courses for students to be successful both in the first two years of medical school and on the MCATs.

Complete all of your medical school prerequisites prior to submitting your application. Although this may not be required, preference may be given to those applicants who have all of their prerequisites completed.

29 Do not assume that you can substitute courses or AP credits for your medical school prerequisites.

Check with each medical school regarding its Advanced Placement (AP) policies. Some medical schools will not accept AP credits to meet any of their medical school prerequisites. Other medical schools may accept the credits, but only if your primary undergraduate college has given you transfer credit and the courses are clearly indicated on your primary college transcript. Other medical schools may require that you take additional upper-level courses at your primary college in the subject area in which your AP credit was earned in order to show that you can handle more rigorous college-level science courses.

If you want to substitute courses that you have taken for the medical school prerequisite courses (e.g., biochemistry in place of organic chemistry), you will need to check with each individual medical school to see which substitutions it will accept, if any. Medical school policies on course substitutions vary.

30 Do not assume that your application is complete.

Be proactive! It is your responsibility to be sure that all of your application materials were received by the medical schools' deadlines. Because of the volume of mail that admissions offices receive, it is best for you to follow up and confirm that each office has everything it needs and that items have arrived on time to complete your application. Do not assume anything or rely on the medical school admissions office to notify you of an incomplete application or problems. By the time you learn what you are missing, it might be too late. Many schools have "applicant status" pages on their Web sites that provide an eassfsy way for you to check to see if your application is complete and to track when materials arrive.

31 Keep your contact information current.

If any of your contact information changes over the course of the admissions process, be sure to update it with AMCAS and with each medical school.

If you are going to pay the money and go through the process of applying, then you want to make sure that you can be reached by the admissions staff if they try to contact you. Make sure that all schools have your correct phone number, current address, and newest e-mail address on file.

Be sure to let the AMCAS know of your changes as well so the schools and the AMCAS have consistent and correct contact information. Try not to invite confusion at any level of the application process.

32 Be a well rounded applicant.

There are many different people on an admissions committee. It is important to keep in mind that each person is looking for something different. That is the beauty of a committee. Some people are looking for students who have spent a great deal of time obtaining clinical experiences, others might be more interested in your research experiences, others in your grades and MCAT scores, and still others in your extracurricular activities during your undergraduate studies.

Your high school counselors probably told you that it was important to get involved and be a well-rounded applicant when applying to undergraduate colleges; now you are hearing it again as you apply to medical school. Once you get to medical school your advisors are going to tell you the same thing in preparation for applying to residency programs.

Admissions committees are eager to see applicants who have something more to offer the student body and the greater community than just good grades. They want to see significant contributions made both inside and outside of the academic arena. They want to see that you will make a difference in the field of medicine.

Letters of Recommendation

Letters of recommendation can be one of the more stressful parts of completing an application, but they can also be one the most important parts. Select your letter writers thoughtfully. Ask individuals who know you well and have insight into your intellectual capabilities and your interpersonal strengths. They should be people who can attest to your motivation, drive, and suitability for a career in medicine.

Selecting the wrong letter writers can really hurt your application. The best letters of recommendation are those that are submitted from a pre-health committee. They should include individual letters or excerpts from faculty, supervisors, and other people who know you well. If your college or university does not have a pre-health committee, letters of recommendation from faculty may be acceptable. Check with each medical school regarding the specific letters they require.

Be sure that all of your letters of recommendation are submitted on letterhead. If they are not they may not be accepted. It is also important that your entire name, including middle name and AAMC ID, be listed on each letter submitted to avoid confusion with another applicant with the same name. You can also help to avoid confusion by reminding your letter writers to use your full name in their letters of recommendation.

Interfolio
www.interfolio.com

Applicants use Interfolio as an online tool to store, manage, and deliver their letters of recommendation to approximately seventy medical schools. Applicants can create an online portfolio at Interfolio and track their letters of recommendation. This makes things much easier for the letter writer, the medical schools, and the applicant.

VirtualEvals
www.virtualevals.org

This electronic service was designed to enhance the efficiency of how letters of recommendation are sent to the admissions offices at medical schools. Letters of recommendation are transmitted electronically from the undergraduate college or university to the admissions office of the colleges to which you are applying. This has allowed the letter of recommendation process to become much more efficient and cost effective.

Applicants do not have access to VirtualEvals. Only the senders and receivers of the letters have access, so it is a very secure way to send letters of recommendation.

Check out their Web site to see what VirtualEvals is all about, what the advantages are, which medical schools participate, which undergraduate schools participate, and how it all started.

Many undergraduate colleges and universities are now using either VirtualEvals or Interfolio online letter of recommendation services to transmit applicants' letters of recommendation to the various medical schools. This is one of the best ways for a medical school to receive your letters of recommendation. This method ensures they will not be lost in the mail, they are downloaded by the medical schools with ease, and applicants can also confirm that they have been received by each medical school.

Check to see if your school utilizes either VirtualEvals or Interfolio and if the medical schools you are applying to accept letters of recommendation via these services.

33 Be sure that your letter writers know you on a personal level.

It is difficult for admissions staff to evaluate letters written by people who do not know the student well. It is not helpful when your letter says, "Jane Doe was a student in my introduction to biology course. She was in the top 10% of her class of 300 students. She did well academically earning a solid 'A' in my course. I think she will be successful in medical school and eventually make a great doctor." A form letter from a department chair will do more harm than a personal letter from an instructor who knows your academic capabilities and your character and is willing to write specifically about you.

It is important that your recommender says something about you that is not obvious in your application. She/he should discuss what kind of person you are, what kind of student you are/were, what you are/were able to offer your classmates, as well as commenting on your character, integrity, drive, and motivation. Therefore, it is imperative that these letters be written by and requested of people who have a solid understanding of you and your desire to enter medical school and pursue a career as a physician.

34 Limit the number of letters of recommendation that you submit.

Every medical school has different requirements, so know what they are. Some schools will not accept more than two letters of recommendation while others will only accept letters from faculty in particular disciplines. If you submit fifteen letters of recommendation, they will not all be read. Admissions committees will select the letters that they think are the most relevant.

35 Make sure your letters of recommendation are relevant.

Do not submit a letter of recommendation from the physician who fixed your broken arm when you were five. An M.D. after your recommender's name does not mean much if he/she does not really know you. Be thoughtful and selective in asking people to write your letters of recommendation.

36 Do not have your parents write a letter of recommendation.

Yes, it really happens. Of course your parents are going to say how wonderful you are; they love you! Admissions committees are looking for letters that describe many different characteristics about you but not what your parents can offer.

37 Do not write your own letters of recommendation and forge someone else's signature.

This seems obvious, but it has been attempted several times. It is very likely that the admissions committee will detect the fraud and then your chances of going to medical school will be gone forever!

Falsifying any part of your application will lead to the automatic rejection of your application.

38 Waive your rights to access your letters of recommendation.

It is in your best interest to waive your rights to your letters of recommendation. If you refuse, admissions committee members may wonder if there is something that you are trying to hide. It also casts doubt on whether your letter writers will be completely open in their assessment of you if you will have access to their letters. Some pre-med advisors, in fact, will not submit a letter of recommendation on the student's behalf if the student has not waived his/her rights. Students may be required to have their letter writers send their letters directly to each of the medical schools.

The Personal Statement

The personal statement or essay is probably one of the most important parts of the application. It really is the only place in the screening process that you actually become you! You need to make yourself stand out and make the reader want to get to know more about you. This is a great place to tell a story about yourself. How did you get to this point? Was there a particular experience that led you to the field of medicine? Was there a particular patient or physician that made you realize that pursuing a career in medicine was the right move for you? Polish your essay in every way possible! Make sure it flows, is written well, and tells the reader exactly what you want it to say about you.

Do not reiterate everything in your application when writing your personal statement. There is no need to talk about your MCAT scores, your GPA, or where you went to undergraduate school. Write about something that makes you special.

Be careful that relevant experiences or activities are not hidden in your personal statement. List these experiences in the experiences section, then discuss specifics about them in your personal statement. Sometimes students discuss their clinical experiences in the personal statement only, and the significance and specifics of the experiences get lost.

The Personal Statement in a Nutshell

❖ Format.
  ➢ Short separated paragraphs.
  ➢ Perfect grammar.
  ➢ Avoid trickiness (screenplay, poems).
❖ Content.
  ➢ Write it for your best friend.
❖ Read it out loud.
  ➢ Is it clear?
❖ Avoid puffery, name dropping, inauthentic quotes.
❖ Tell a story.
❖ Be honest but avoid confusion.

Thank you to E. Gregory Keating

---

39 Do not quote Robert Frost in your personal statement.

Be original. Quotes from Robert Frost are very popular on medical school applications. You should probably leave him out of the process. You can be serious or use humor, but just be creative, original, and yourself.

One student began his essay by comparing the different roles of ants in an ant colony to the role of a health professional. By the end of the essay, not only had he built a convincing point for the similarities, but his creative approach had made his application stand out among the other applications.

Another non-traditional applicant began by stating how his responsibilities as a reference librarian for the past eleven years were similar to the responsibilities of a physician. Again, this made the reader pause to ask what similarities could possibly exist between these two very different positions? By the end of the essay he had demonstrated, using humor and creativity, that his experiences had helped him develop the strengths necessary to become a dedicated medical student and eventually a physician. At the same time he was able to convey all the reasons why he was applying to medical school as a non-traditional student and what it was about him that made him "special."

40 Use spellcheck and proofread your entire application.

Spellcheck will not pick up words used incorrectly, poor grammar, or run-on sentences. Proofread your personal statement very carefully. Read your essay, reread your essay, then reread your essay again. Does it make sense to you? Allow some time to lapse in between rereadings. If you read your essay twelve times in the same day you will miss obvious errors. Let a day or two pass and then revisit your essay again. This will allow you to look at it with a fresh perspective.

Have someone else read your personal statement, preferably someone who does not know you very well. Does it make sense to him/her? Does she/he get a good sense of who you are and the message you are trying to convey? Keep in mind that this is the only part of the application where you really have the opportunity to individualize yourself outside of your numbers. Will the reader be left with a strong impression of who you are, what you are all about, and your suitability for a career in medicine?

41 If you are applying to medical school and you want to be a physician be sure to spell "physician" correctly.

"Physician," "pediatrician," "orthopedic surgeon" ... If you want to be one, be sure you know how to spell it if you want to avoid the "no thank you" pile.

42 When putting together your personal statement do not generalize or criticize all doctors.

Do not forget that physicians will be reviewing your application; therefore it is a bad strategy to suggest that most physicians are incompetent and you are going to be the ideal doctor and rescue our health care system.

Gimme a Break!
You Might Want to Reconsider
Your Personal Statement!

➤ "The possibility that I might discover a drug that could revolutionize medicine, coupled with my love for learning is why I have chosen to pursue research this semester."

➤ "I was able to overcome this mentally and emotionally stressful point in my life due to my undeterred and undying passion for a career in medicine."

➤ "While volunteering at my local hospital, I often had a gut-wrenching feeling of helplessness."

➤ "Suddenly I heard the crunch of metal against bone, and blood spattered everywhere. Everyone lost their heads in the ensuing moments except me. Thanks to my cool-headed actions, we were able to get our neighbor's dog to the vet in time."

Thank you to E. Gregory Keating

---

43 Be careful not to start every sentence in your essay or personal statement with "I."

Admissions committees want to learn about you, but be careful that it does not sound like bragging. There is a fine line between confidence and overconfidence or cockiness. A narrative about some experience you have had might make your application stand out, but be careful not to over inflate the importance of what you have done. Be honest and modest.

44 Keep your essay clear and well organized.

An essay with no breaks or paragraphs is hard to read, especially when yours might be one among several hundred that an admissions officer might be reading or reviewing in an afternoon. Always be conscious of how things will look to the person who is evaluating your application. If your essay is difficult to read or poorly organized, it may get overlooked.

45 Watch profanity in your personal statement.

Admissions committees actually do read personal statements. They are a really important aspect of an application. Quoting a profanity in a pertinent personal story can be risky. What seems to you to be a vivid recreation could actually offend some members of the admissions committee. Why take that chance?

You know the words to avoid, but do not forget the more common slang words that do not sound very professional: "sucks," "bastard," "dude," or "awesome."

Experiences — Clinical, Research, Volunteer, and Extracurricular Activities

It is important that you choose the above activities carefully. Not only are admissions committees looking for academically qualified students, but they are also looking for students who are self-motivated and dedicated to serving others. They are seeking compassionate, caring, and honest students who possess high ethical standards and can effectively manage their time.

By getting involved in a variety of different experiences you are showing the admissions committee that you are able to handle multiple activities at once, all the while maintaining a solid academic performance. It is important to show the admissions committee that you can successfully balance your school work with all of your outside activities. This will help them evaluate your ability to handle the demands of your life as a physician. Most medical schools are looking for a combination of clinical experiences, in which you shadow physicians and have patient contact, extracurricular activities and leadership opportunities, community service or volunteer work, and research experiences.

What About Those Extracurricular Activities?

➤ Name the activity, your role in it, and the depth of your involvement.
➤ Few and intense vs. many "boutique" contacts.
➤ Direct patient contact.
➤ Cite non-medical service as well.
➤ Catalogue them honestly.

Thank you to E. Gregory Keating

---

46 Do not try to impress the admissions committee with everything you have ever done in your entire life.

Things that you did during junior high are probably not necessary at this level. If you want the admissions committee to know of your longstanding interest in being a physician, your personal statement is probably the best place for this.

47 Adequately describe each activity and experience.

Do not simply list your activities like you would on a resume. Elaborate on your experiences and make clear to the reader how this activity might be relevant to your success in medical school. Do not leave out pertinent information regarding each of your experiences. Highlight all your responsibilities and what you got out of each experience.

48 Get involved in extracurricular activities on your college campus, but be careful not to "pad" your resume with the things you think the committee wants to see.

Be careful that you are not selecting activities just because you think they will look good on your application. Leadership roles are very important. Spend a significant amount of time doing things you enjoy and do them well. Admissions committees are looking for quality over quantity. Find a balance that you are comfortable with that combines academics, extracurricular activities, work, and family. No one wants you to give up your entire life to prepare for your medical school application, so continue doing things that are important to you.

49 Remember that there are only 168 hours in a week.

Be sure that when you are adding up your school work, class time, extracurricular activities, shadowing, and research experiences, that they do not add up to more than 168 hours. Be realistic, truthful, and accurate when filling out your activities page. If you have a lot of activities and your grades have suffered as a result of overextending yourself, this will not work in your favor.

50 Being a bridesmaid is not an extracurricular activity ...

... and surfing the Web is not a hobby. Be careful about the impression that activities like this will make on members of the admissions committee. They are looking for substantial, quality experiences that tell them something about who you are and the things that you are passionate about. The activities that you list should reflect your interests and serve as a possible indicator of how committed you are to service work, how well you work with others, and how well you manage your time.

51 Giving blood once a year is not a volunteer activity.

If you consider giving blood once a year a volunteer activity, you had better get out there and get some additional volunteer experiences. Although this is a good start, it really does not say enough about your dedication to serving others and your drive to be a physician. It is viewed as "the right thing to do," but is not going to be enough to prove your dedication to serving others.

What Should Your Activities Convey?

➤ I like to serve people. I can do this day after day.
➤ I have given medicine a good try, and I think I understand its joys and trials.

Thank you to E. Gregory Keating

---

52 Timing is essential.

It is important that your experiences and activities be an ongoing process. Do not start your extracurricular experiences right before applying to medical school. This will be viewed as simply getting the experiences because you have to, instead of doing them because of your own interest or desire.

53 Clinical experience is absolutely necessary.

You need to show the admissions committee that you have investigated the field of medicine and are sure that you know exactly what you are getting yourself into. It is important that you have a clear understanding of what a physician does during the day, and how they interact with their patients, families of their patients, and other health professionals.

If you indicate that you are leaning toward a certain specialty, for example, pediatric orthopedic surgery, be prepared to discuss what you know about this specialty during your interview. Be able to discuss what you have observed, the day-to-day responsibilities of a pediatric orthopedic surgeon, the types of patients they usually see, and why you think you might enjoy this specialty area.

If you always thought you might enjoy being an oncologist or an otolaryngologist, then shadow physicians in these areas, in addition to those in other areas, to experience a variety of roles and responsibilities. This exploration will not only help you decide that medicine is the right career for you, but will also help you to convey better in your personal statement and/or interview your reasons for wanting to enter the medical profession.

If you happen to be the child of a physician, it is important that you get out and get additional clinical experiences of shadowing other physicians and getting patient contact. This will show the admissions committee that this is something that **you** want and have investigated on your own, not simply something that you have heard your parent discuss at the dinner table.

54 Tell the truth!

Everything in your application is "fair game." If you listed it, be prepared to talk about it during an interview. Admissions committee members have been known to call the "contact person" whom you list in your experiences. Be sure that you have done what you say you have done. If you are in the process of founding an organization, say that. Do not say you already founded it, only to have a member of the admissions committee check with your undergraduate college and find that the organization does not yet exist.

55 Service volunteer work is very important.

Countless students have said that they are interested in the field of medicine because they want to help people. If this is why you are going into medicine, be sure that your application contains evidence that you have helped people. Being a physician means that you will be dedicating your life to serving others. You need to be sure you want this.

One way to convey your commitment to service work is by volunteering and trying to make a difference in your community. Volunteer for Hospice, become a literacy volunteer or a Big Brother or Big Sister. Get out there, get involved, and make a difference!

56 Research experiences are not required at every medical school, so investigate which schools require or recommend research.

Some schools do require research. They think that it is a very important part of the medical profession and is the foundation for medical knowledge. Over the course of your career, you will need to utilize various forms of medical literature to treat your future patients and remain current in your field.

It is important for you to apply to schools that are consistent with your own interest, or lack of interest, in research. Do not do research just because you think you have to; do it because you really want to do it.

If you have done research, be prepared to talk about it. You will need to be able to describe your project in detail and discuss exactly what role you played in the research.

If you are unable to describe and/or explain your research, your duties, and your findings, then the admissions committee will be left wondering if this is a case of embellishment. If you have simply done research for the sake of having it look good on a medical school application, this will be easily detected.

You also may want to explore non-scientific research as well. This could be a great opportunity to show independent thinking, an appreciation for the process of research, and a slant toward lifelong learning without being limited to working with pipettes!

The Interview Process

You got the call, and you have a medical school interview. Now what? The interview can truly make or break an applicant. The committee saw something that they liked in your application and wants to learn more about you, find out what you have to offer the field of medicine, and to see if their medical school is the right "fit" for you. Be kind, courteous, respectful, and professional to everyone you come into contact with. Prepare for your interviews and do your homework on each medical school. Practice your interviews, but not to the point where your answers sound rehearsed. Prepare questions to ask your interviewers, review your AMCAS application, and keep in mind that you are evaluating the medical schools just as much as they are evaluating you.

If you are traveling a long distance for several interviews, it is acceptable to contact the admissions offices at the schools and let them know you will be in the area during a particular time and would be happy to come in for an interview. If the school will be granting you an interview, they may be able to grant your request, saving you time and money.

The Medical School Interview

➢ Think of the person you talk with the best.
➢ Have some explanations, but do not overpractice.
➢ Do not criticize; do not make excuses.
➢ Do not be drawn into being an expert ... if you are not.
➢ This is not confession.

Thank you to E. Gregory Keating

57

It is not necessary to wear a black suit, white shirt, and red tie.

It is important to dress professionally, but spice it up a bit and be a little different. With that said, be careful not to be too casual or too revealing in your attire. Women should wear a pantsuit or skirt and blouse. Men should wear a suit or khakis and sports jacket with a shirt and tie.

58

Get enough sleep and be well rested for your interview.

It is important to be at your best during your interview. Applicants have actually fallen asleep during group interviews and then awakened to ask a question that was already covered. If necessary, get up, walk out, and compose yourself rather than embarrassing yourself by nodding off.

59 Do not go out and get "smashed" the night before your interview.

If you happen to have friends in the area of your interview and get together the night before your interview, try to keep it low key. If you do go out for a night on the town, be sure not to talk about the previous night's events in great detail with your interviewer or within earshot of the admissions director or a member of the admissions staff.

60 If your interviewer says something inappropriate or creates an uncomfortable interview situation for you, tell the admissions director.

If you do not tell the admissions director, he/she will never know that an interviewer is not behaving appropriately. It is important that you speak up before a decision has been made on your application, as decisions are often final. After you have been waitlisted or rejected, your concerns may seem less valid. Let the admissions director know about your concerns prior to leaving on interview day. Once you leave there may not be anything that can be done to help you or to rectify the situation.

Possible Questions to Ask During Your Interview

➤ Please describe the medical school curriculum. (Is it problem-based? Organ-based?)
➤ Are the lectures taped?
➤ Is there a note-taking service?
➤ Is a PDA or laptop required?
➤ Can you tell me about the international opportunities available? (Summers and electives?)
➤ Is there patient contact in the first year?
➤ Can you tell me about the research opportunities for students?
➤ What is the grading system like? (Pass/fail? Modified A/B/C?)
➤ Is this a very competitive environment?
➤ Are there support services available? (Personal counseling, tutoring, advising?)
➤ Are the match statistics available?
➤ May I send updated materials for the admissions committee to consider?
➤ Are there any special programs that this medical school is known for?
➤ How do students perform on the boards?
➤ How accessible are the faculty?
➤ How are students evaluated during their clinical years?
➤ Are their extracurricular activities available?
➤ Is a car necessary for clinical rotations?
➤ Are students allowed to participate on medical school committees?
➤ Are students involved in community service projects, either required or voluntary?
➤ What made you choose to complete your medical education here?
➤ What made you decide to work here?
➤ What do you think the school's greatest strengths are?
➤ What do you see changing here over the next four years?

61 Always come to your interview prepared with questions for your interviewers.

If you have two interviewers and the first one answered your questions, ask again; another perspective is always helpful. If you have no questions, you could be viewed as being uninterested in the institution. Medical schools want to accept applicants that want to be there and are enthusiastic about their program and institution.

This is your opportunity to learn more about the medical school in order to help you decide whether or not it is the right "fit" for you. Can you see yourself there? Would you be happy there if accepted? Does the school offer the social and academic experiences that you are looking for in your medical education?

Do not, however, pepper your interviewers with questions that could easily be answered by viewing the school's Web site or from the materials you received. Your questions need to be genuine and should come naturally out of the conversation.

62 Do not try to be someone that you are not.

Most experienced interviewers can detect an insincere applicant. Interviews are designed to get to know who you are and to see if this particular medical school is the right medical school for you. Relax and be yourself.

63 If you are running late for your interview, be sure to call.

If you are caught in traffic, lost, or have missed a flight, be sure to call the admissions office and let them know. Most interview days are carefully planned and schedules can be pretty tight. There may not be a lot of wiggle room. Make sure to apologize if you are late so that the staff knows you are taking this interview seriously.

Sometimes students become lax about their responsibilities when they already have an acceptance but are still interviewing. If you are really not interested in being there, cancel your interview as early as humanly possible. There are many other students who would be happy to take your interview spot.

64 Dress for the weather.

Do some homework on the climate where you will be interviewing. For instance, when applicants are interviewing in the month of January in Central New York, chances are they will need coats, hats, gloves, boots, and/or an umbrella.

You never know how far you may have to walk for your interviews, campus tour, or parking. You do not want to show up at your interview late, wet, and shivering because you just trudged up a slush-covered hill in a skirt or dress shoes.

65 Turn off your cell phones.

If you must leave your cell phone on, put it on vibrate. You do not want some kind of funky ring tone like Kanye West's "Gold Digger," Beyonce's "Irreplaceable," or Justin Timberlake's "SexyBack," going off during your interview. That would be embarrassing and inappropriate.

66 If you do keep your phone on, be polite.

Use common sense and good phone etiquette. If you must answer your phone while in the presence of an admissions staff member, do not hold up your finger and tell her/him to wait for you so that you can take the call. Tell the caller you will get back to them as soon as possible, and apologize to the person you have left waiting. Remember, everything you do in the interview process reflects what you might be doing to a patient or colleague.

67 Be prepared to talk about your institutional action(s).

The admissions committee will want to know as much as they can about any institutional action against you. Alcohol offenses, plagiarism, and academic probation seem to be the most common violations. Plagiarism offenses and alcohol violations have become more common over the past couple of years. All such actions are serious and need to be addressed with sincerity in your application. Several similar violations may be seen as a cause for concern and may affect how strongly your application is considered. Anticipate these areas of concern regarding your prior institutional action(s) and think about how you are going to explain and account for your actions in the best possible light. Remember to be honest and sincere in your explanation.

68 Be prepared to talk about pass/fail courses, withdrawing from courses, or repeating courses.

Interviews are the perfect opportunity for the admissions committee to get answers to questions that they have about your academic past. What they are looking for is clarification of any "red flags" that they see in your academic record. Be honest. Avoid blaming anyone. Focus on the positive, for example, what you have learned from the experience and how you have applied what you learned to the success of your future studies.

Be very careful in your explanations. Perhaps you withdrew from organic chemistry because you were taking a heavy course load and wanted to take it when you had a lighter schedule, and perhaps increase your chances of earning an "A." This may indicate to an interviewer that you are not up for the challenge of the medical school curriculum. It is also not a good idea to say you dropped a class because the professor was difficult and you wanted to take it the next semester with an "easier" professor.

69 Do not give "canned" answers to interview questions.

Interviewers are looking for genuine answers to their questions. So do not answer their questions with answers that you think they want to hear.

There might not always be a right or wrong answer to a question posed during an interview. The interview has more to do with how you express yourself than with what you say. Sometimes applicants may give an answer to a question that they *wanted* the interviewer to ask rather than answering what was actually asked. This may call an applicant's listening skills into question. Ask for clarification if you do not understand the question.

Be sure to review your answers to the medical school's secondary application as part of your interview preparation. If you are asked a question about an answer that you gave in your application and you respond with "I have no idea what you are talking about. Can I see the essay?", you will sound shallow and unprepared.

70 Practice your interviews.

Try doing some mock interviews with someone at your career center or someone you do not know very well so that you are a little uncomfortable. It is important that you interview well, but it is equally important not to sound rehearsed. If you do not know the answer to a particular question, it is okay to say that you do not know, but do your best to answer the question. The interviewer may not be looking for the "right" answer, but they may be interested in seeing how you handle yourself or how you think.

You need to be able to answer basic questions. For instance, if you are asked what your three greatest strengths are, you need three, not two. You can find examples of frequently asked medical school interview questions online. You can also visit <www.StudentDoctor.net> to view questions that other applicants were asked during their interviews. This preparation will help you to anticipate some of the questions you may be asked.

Possible Interview Questions

➢ Tell me about yourself.
➢ What do you do in your spare time?
➢ How would your friends describe you?
➢ How did you select your undergraduate institution?
➢ How did you select your major?
➢ What undergraduate science class was your favorite and why?
➢ What kinds of non-science courses have you taken, and how will you apply your experiences in those classes to a career in medicine?
➢ What are your strengths (both academically and personally)?
➢ What exposure have you had to the medical field?
➢ Why do you want to be a doctor?
➢ What have you done to solidify that medicine is the right career for you?
➢ Why makes you think you would be a good doctor?
➢ Describe your research/clinical/volunteer experiences in medicine.
➢ What are you looking for in a medical school?
➢ What is it specifically about our medical school that made you want to apply?
➢ What will you do if you are not accepted to medical school?
➢ If you were not accepted to medical school, what other profession would you pursue?
➢ If accepted to medical school, what do you think will be the greatest challenge in completing it?
➢ How would you contribute to the student body here?
➢ What sets you apart from other applicants?

More Possible Interview Questions

➢ How would you deal with another medical professional who holds differing views from yours?
➢ What do you consider the biggest problem in healthcare today? How will you address it in your future career?
➢ Where do you see yourself in ten years?
➢ Why should we accept you?
➢ What would you identify as weaknesses in your application?
➢ What should I tell the admissions committee about you?
➢ What personal accomplishment are you most proud of?
➢ Who is your role model and why? How has that person inspired you to be who you are today?
➢ Do you have any questions for me?

---

71 Do not answer your interviewer's questions with one-word answers.

You must elaborate on your answers. The admissions committee wants to know as much as they can about you. It is important for you to demonstrate clearly your ability to articulate your thoughts and to communicate effectively. Effective communication skills are crucial when working with patients and as part of a team with other health professionals.

72 Send a thank-you note to your interviewers.

If you really enjoyed your interview experience, send a thank-you note to your interviewer(s) or student host. A personal handwritten card, a typed letter, or an e-mail are all acceptable ways to show your appreciation. If you do send a thank-you note, be sure that you send it to the right person at the right medical school.

73 Do not tell your interviewers that their school is not your first choice.

You must be able to say something special about a particular program or school and what it was that made you want to apply there.

Take a brief moment and look over the curriculum or special programs offered, and find something specific that appeals to you and your interests. You will be better able to convey interest in a program (even if it is not your "top choice") if you have taken some time to research the program that you are applying to. With a limited number of seats available, why would a school want to award a seat to someone who does not really want to be there?

74 Answer honestly if an interviewer asks where else you have interviewed.

Try not to get defensive or paranoid if you are asked this question. Many times the interviewers are just curious to see which other medical schools you are considering. It will not be used against you. You do not necessarily have to name the names of the other medical schools; instead talk about the qualities you are most looking for in a medical school. It gives the interviewer a sense of what you are looking for in a medical school, and why. What was/is important to you? Are you looking for an urban/rural setting? What is the patient population? Are there opportunities for service work or research? Are you looking for a curriculum that allows you the flexibility to experience and pursue a variety of interests? Do you prefer an organ-based or problem-based approach?

75 Do not bring your parents or significant other with you to your interview.

The interview process should demonstrate your independence and maturity. You do not want to stand out among the other applicants in this way and be remembered as the applicant that brought his/her mom along.

76 Sit in on classes.

Sitting in on classes is critically important. Not only will you learn how the classes are taught, but you can observe the dynamics between the faculty and the students and among the students themselves. How do the students interact with one another and with their professors? Does the environment appear to be cutthroat or supercompetitive? Is the faculty interested in the material they are presenting? Do they seem approachable? Do class interactions fit with the environment you are looking for? Do the students appear to be happy? Your day on campus is your opportunity to determine whether or not the school is the right "fit" for you.

77 Ask current students about their experiences.

See if you can spend the night before your interview with a current student; he or she is your best resource! Not only can this save you money, but it is also a great way to learn more about a school. Contact the admissions office in advance. They often can put you in touch with students who have volunteered to host applicants the night before their interviews.

When you attend your interview days, make the most of being on the medical school's campus. Look around, sit in on classes, check out the library, hang out in the cafeteria, sit in the student lounge, walk around the campus, and most importantly, talk to students. They have been where you are and know what you are going through, and they are often happy to share their personal experiences with prospective students.

Questions To Ask Current Students

➤ What do they like about the medical school?
➤ Are there things they do not like?
➤ Why did they choose this particular medical school?
➤ Is it competitive or cutthroat?
➤ Are they happy here?
➤ What makes the school stand out?
➤ How accessible is the faculty?
➤ Are there any special programs?
➤ What is the town or city like?
➤ What have their clinical experiences been like?
➤ When did they first have patient contact?
➤ What is the curriculum like?
➤ Are they happy with the curriculum?
➤ What kind of residency planning is available?
➤ Is there counseling, tutoring, and other assistance available?
➤ Do they recommend the support services?

---

78 Do not badmouth the school you are applying to when staying overnight with current students.

Keep in mind that there is always some type of evaluation process taking place even if it is informal or "off the record." Always be polite and respectful. Student hosts are taking you in and allowing you to stay in their home, sometimes while they are studying for exams. When applying to a medical school, you are *asking* them to honor your request for admission. Entry into medical school is a *privilege* and not a right, no matter how outstanding an applicant's grades or experiences are.

79 Bring a book.

Chances are there will be down time during your interview day, so be prepared to wait. For some of you it will be too much time; for others of you it will not be enough time. It is difficult to make everyone happy. Bring a book along and if you have too much down time you can catch up on some pleasure reading. If you are asked the question, "What is the last book you read?", you will be able to provide a quick answer.

80 Watch how you shake hands.

Be confident, look your interviewer in the eye, and do not worry if your hands are sweaty because you are nervous. That is a lot better than a limp handshake and a passive or insecure appearance.

81 Be sure to bring extra cash on your interview day.

Always plan on a little more money than you think you might need for incidentals such as parking, taxis, porters, and food. It is embarrassing to have to borrow money from the dean of admissions to get your car out of the parking garage.

82 Eat breakfast.

Catch the continental breakfast at your hotel on your interview day. Most medical schools do not serve breakfast and it may be a while before you are served lunch. Eating breakfast will also help to wake you up and have a clear mind for your interviews.

83 Do not complain about the lunch you are served at your interview.

If you have specific restrictions (e.g., kosher, vegetarian, etc.) be sure to notify the medical school at least one week prior to your interview day. Many schools have their lunches catered and must place their orders several days in advance.

84 Do not be too casual in your interview.

Some interviewers take a formal approach to interviewing, while others might prefer to be more conversational in their approach. Even if an interviewer takes a more laid back approach, remember that you are **still** being interviewed and that you are applying to a professional school. Do not lean back in your chair and put your feet up on the table. Interviewers do not want to hear about how you like to "chill" in your free time and "kick it" with your friends.

85 When asked about end-of-life issues, respond with appropriate dignity.

Do not say "I don't have a problem with dead people," or "It's good to tell jokes to lighten the mood."

Death is an issue you will no doubt have to confront as a physician. How will you handle losing a patient? Are you comfortable with death? What experience, if any, do you have with death? How do you feel about a patient's right to die? Or euthanasia? Reflect on these questions and know where you stand on these topics. You may also be asked some tough ethical questions during your interview.

86 Be prepared for interview day surprises.

Ask questions about the different interview days at each medical school before your interviews. Talk to your pre-health advisor and check out the medical school Web site, such as the interview feedback section on <www.studentdoctor.net>.

Talk to other students who have interviewed where you are interviewing. It is important to know how the interviews are structured and conducted. Will there be stress interviews, surprise essays, panel interviews, student interviewers? Which components of your application will each of your interviewers have? Will it be a closed file interview, where your interviewer does not have any information about you other than your name?

87 If you can, find out in advance who will be interviewing you.

You may not know who is interviewing you until the morning you arrive on campus. If a computer is available and you can find out who will be interviewing you, you can use some of your down time to learn about your interviewer on the college Web site. Your extra effort could make you stand out and might also reveal some common interests between you and your interviewer.

88 Do not panic if your interviewer does not ask every question there is to ask about you.

Interviews are mostly designed to recruit students. If you feel that something very relevant to your candidacy was overlooked, or you want to add something that was not covered in your interview, it may be appropriate to submit a follow-up letter to the admissions committee. At the end of your interview, you may also ask your interviewer to share a particular piece of information with the admissions committee.

Overall, let the interviewer control the interview and the flow of conversation. Perhaps your interviewer loves opera and you are an accomplished singer. It is okay if the interview centers around that interest. Most interviewers are trying to gain a sense of your overall maturity, intelligence, compassion, and depth. An experienced interviewer can assess all of these things by asking questions that are other than medically related.

89 Try to relax enough to be interested in your interviewer.

This may help you to get out of your own head and in turn may reduce your anxiety. Who is this person? What does she/he do? How does he/she view the institution? How long has she/he been here? How can his/her experience shed light on the institution and on your understanding about whether it might be a good fit for you?

Your ability to demonstrate interest in your interviewer could be seen as a surrogate for the interest you will eventually have in your patients. The ability to meet a stranger and engage in an open, mutually satisfying dialogue demonstrates good potential for doctoring, a profession where you need to meet strangers and establish rapport quickly on a daily basis.

90 If you have the opportunity to interview with a current student, do it!

Current students can offer you some really great insight into the college and into medical school life. They have been through this challenging process and are now living the life of a medical student. They are often very willing to discuss their experiences, decisions and even regrets, and to give their honest opinions about the program they have chosen. Student interviewers are usually not paid, and volunteer their time to help the admissions office select the best applicants for the next year's entering class.

Student interviewers tend to look at prospective students very differently. They seem to assess students more as potential colleagues than as potential medical students. They may eventually be working alongside you and referring patients to you.

91 Do not leave the interview day early.

Leaving before the campus tour sends a bad message about your level of interest in attending the medical school you are visiting. Not only are medical schools looking for the most qualified students, but also students who want to be there. It costs time and money to travel around the country and attend each interview for medical school, so why not relax and find out as much as you can about each school?

Be sure to plan your travel according to the interview schedule at the medical school. Do not show up the morning of your interview and tell the admissions staff that you need to leave by noon to catch a flight, when you have a 1:30 interview. Making the admissions office scramble to accommodate your schedule is not the way you want to be remembered.

92 Be conscious of your nonverbal behaviors during the interview.

Look your interviewer in the eye. Eye contact, facial expressions, posture, and hand gestures are all incredibly important! It is also important to keep in mind a person's personal space.

Top Five Nonverbals for Interviewing

According to <collegegrad.com>, many interviews fail because of lack of proper communication. But communication is more than just what you say. Often it is the nonverbal communication that we are least aware of, yet speaks the loudest. Following are the top five nonverbals, ranked in order of importance, when it comes to interviewing:

➢ **Eye Contact** — Unequaled in importance! If you have a habit of looking away while listening, it shows lack of interest and a short attention span. If you fail to maintain eye contact while speaking, it might show a lack of confidence or send a subtle indication that you may be lying. Don't just assume you have good eye contact. Ask. Watch. Practice. Ask others if you ever lack proper eye contact. If so was it during speaking or listening? Sit down with a friend and practice until you are comfortable maintaining sincere, continuous eye contact.

Top Five Nonverbals
for Interviewing (continued)

➤ **Facial Expressions** — Take a good, long, hard look at yourself in the mirror. Look at yourself as others would. Do you look scared? Bored? Engaged? Add a simple feature that nearly every interviewee forgets – smile! A true and genuine smile says you are a happy person and delighted to be interviewing today.

➤ **Posture** — Posture sends a signal of confidence. Stand tall, walk tall, and most of all, sit tall. When you are seated, make sure you sit at the front edge of the chair, slightly leaning forward, intent on the subject at hand.

➤ **Gestures** — Gestures should be limited during the interview. Do not use artificial gestures to heighten the importance of the issue at hand. You will merely come off as theatrical. When you do use gestures, make sure they are sincere and meaningful.

➤ **Space** — Recognize the boundaries of your personal space and that of others. If you are typical of most Americans, it will range between 30 and 36 inches. Be prepared, however, not to back up or move away from someone who has a personal space that is smaller than your own. Hang in there, take a deep breath, and stand your ground. For most of us, being aware of our personal space is enough to prompt us to stand firm. If you have a smaller than average personal space, make sure you keep your distance so that you do not intimidate someone who needs more room.

WELCH — 101 TIPS

93 Be flexible! Try not to get too irritated if there is a last-minute change during your interview day.

A day in the life of a physician is unpredictable and you often have to deal with less than perfect situations where patients and colleagues do inconvenient things at very inconvenient times. Do not complain!

94 Do not tell your interviewer you are going into medicine for prestige or money.

If that is why you want to be a doctor, then you should find a new profession. There are people who work much less and make much more. You can make more money as an investment banker and usually incur less debt. A career in medicine will be a long, lonely, and hard road if you are in it for the wrong reasons!

Waiting for a Response

It can seem to take forever when you are waiting for an admissions decision. Most medical schools cannot begin sending out admissions decisions until October 15. If you interview in early September, a month and a half is a long wait.

Be sure to ask the following questions during your interview day: How long until a decision is made? How will you hear from the admissions committee, by a status page on the school Web site, by phone call, e-mail, or through the mail? If you are put on a waitlist how does the alternate list work? Are students reevaluated? Is the list ranked? Can you send in new information? If you are denied admission, is there advisement available? Often, your interviewer will not know the answers to these questions, but the admissions staff and director will certainly be able to help you.

95 Be patient!

Chances are you will not hear from an admissions committee for four to six weeks after your interview, in some cases, even longer than that.

96 Do not contact your interviewers to find out "what went wrong" if you are denied admission.

Sometimes medical school interviewers are not members of the medical school admissions committee, and while they do offer their recommendations to the committee, they may not be present or part of the actual voting process when the decision on an application is made. The committee looks at the big picture and takes everything into account — grades and MCAT scores, extracurricular activities, clinical exposure, research experience, work-related experience, letters of recommendation, interviewer ratings, and the competitiveness of the applicant pool that year. To find out how to strengthen your application it is probably best to talk to your pre-health advisor or a member of the medical school admissions staff, if the school offers such advisement.

97 Take advantage of any "Second Visit Day" opportunities at the medical schools to which you have been accepted.

"Second Visit" or "Second Look" days are great opportunities to revisit the medical schools you are truly interested in. This time you will be seriously evaluating what the medical school has to offer you, what makes it unique, and whether it is the right "fit" for you. Since you are no longer being evaluated, this visit should be much more relaxed and you can evaluate the school through different eyes. This visit may be a good time to bring your parents, spouse, or significant other to have them help you evaluate your options. Dress comfortably and leave your suit at home, but be sure to check to see if there is a particular dress code for different events that you might be attending.

Reapplying

Do not reapply unless you have spent adequate time making significant changes to your application. These changes usually come in the form of new grades, MCAT scores, experiences, different letters of recommendation, and/or a new personal statement. This will take a great deal of preparation and is not something that can be accomplished in just a month or so.

First, go back and talk to your pre-health advisor and seek his/her advice about what you should do differently for your next round of applications. Second, while not all medical schools offer application counseling to applicants, if you have the opportunity to meet with an admissions person and go over your application, do it. They are the people reviewing your application and can best point out the strengths and weaknesses of your application. Do not assume that you know what the problem was with your application. It may be something entirely different than what you suspect.

If you were interviewed and later rejected, ask for *honest* feedback from the admissions staff at one or more of the medical schools that interviewed you. If you are able to speak to a member of the admissions staff, do not become defensive. It is important that you take their comments seriously. If you received multiple interviews that resulted in waitlists or post-interview rejections, chances are that your interviews are your weak point and you should improve this skill before interviewing for a second time.

98 Do not, under any circumstances, resubmit the same application.

Make positive changes to your application. If it did not work the first time, chances are that same application is not going to work the second time. Most medical schools will keep application records for a couple of years, and if an applicant resubmits exactly the same application, particularly the same personal statement or letters of recommendation, it will probably be rejected because there is nothing new to evaluate.

How motivated could someone be to become a physician if he/she could not even take the time to write a new personal statement or to request current letters of recommendation? The admissions staff wants to know what you have done to strengthen your application since last applying and they will be looking for changes and improvements in your qualifications. How has the past year or years served to increase your drive and motivation to become a physician?

99 If poor grades were the biggest problem with your previous application, do not reapply until you have nearly finished a post-baccalaureate or graduate program.

If you reapply as soon as you enter the program there will not be enough time to show the admissions committee that you can handle a rigorous science curriculum or graduate-level coursework. Besides, it is unlikely that your grades will be available in time for the admissions committee to consider them.

In some cases, one semester of post-baccalaureate or graduate coursework may not be enough to overcome a previous poor academic record. It is best to relax, do well, and take some time to prove your academic ability and consistency to the admissions committee.

100 Do not assume that because you were on a school's waitlist or alternate list last year, you have a better chance of gaining acceptance this year.

Each year's applicant pool is different from the year before, and most schools will look at applicants independently from year to year. In addition, medical schools may be looking for different things each year when reviewing applications. Think of every application and every interview as a new opportunity to sell yourself to the medical school.

Alternate List

If you are placed on a medical school's alternate or waitlist, call to see if they will accept any additional information from you for further review of your application. You may want to touch base with the medical school to see how their list is moving and to let them know you are still interested in attending should an opening arise. Be sure to have your correct contact information on file.

Many schools will not release much information regarding the movement of their alternate lists. They may tell you generic information such as that you are in the top third, middle third, or bottom third, but they may not tell you how many students are on their list. Some will keep an active alternate list up until the first day of orientation.

Most Importantly ...

101 Always, always be yourself!

Applying to medical school is a very long and often overwhelming process. Applicants can sometimes get caught up in the "They have to like me" or "I will do whatever it takes" attitude to gain acceptance to medical school. It is very important that you are always true to yourself, from your thoughts about pursuing a career in medicine, to your application, to your interview.

Be the person you are, instead of the person you think the medical school is looking for. Every school is different, but you need to go where you feel most comfortable. Choose a school that is the right "fit" for you.

Contact Information for Each Medical School

Following is a complete list of contact information for all 125 medical schools in the United States. It is important to check with each individual medical school to get the most accurate information, as each medical school is different.

Included are the mailing address, phone number, e-mail address, and Web site for each medical school. At the time of publication, to the best of our knowledge, all of this information was up-to-date and accurate. This information may change over time.

An asterisk * indicates that the school participates with the American Medical College Application Service (AMCAS).

ALABAMA

University of Alabama*
    School of Medicine, Office of Student Admissions
    VH 100, 1530 3rd Avenue South
    Birmingham, Alabama 35294-1150
    Phone: (205) 934-2433
    E-mail: medschool@uab.edu
    Web site: www.uab.edu/uasom/

University of South Alabama*
    College of Medicine, Office of Admissions, 2015 MSB
    Mobile, Alabama 36688-0002
    Phone: (251) 460-7176
    E-mail: mscott@usouthal.edu
    Web site: www.southalabama.edu/com/

ARIZONA

University of Arizona*
    College of Medicine
    Admissions Office, P.O. Box 245075
    Tucson, Arizona 85724-5075
    Phone: (520) 626-6214
    E-mail: admissions@medicine.arizona.edu
    Web site: www.medicine.arizona.edu

University of Arkansas*
> College of Medicine, Office of the Dean
> 4301 West Markham Street, Slot 551
> Little Rock, Arkansas 72205-7199
> Phone: (501) 686-5354
> E-mail: southtomg@uams.edu
> Web site: www.uams.edu/com

Loma Linda University*
> School of Medicine, Office of Admissions
> Loma Linda, California 92350
> Phone: (909) 558-4467
> E-mail: admissions.sm@llu.edu
> Web site: www.llu.edu/llu/medicine

Stanford University*
> School of Medicine, Office of Admissions
> 251 Campus Drive, MSOB X3C01
> Stanford, California 94305-5404
> Phone: (650) 723-6861
> E-mail: mdadmissions@stanford.edu
> Web site: med.stanford.edu

University of California - Davis*
> School of Medicine
> Office of Admissions, One Shields Avenue
> Davis, California 95616-8661
> Phone: (530) 752-2717
> E-mail: medadmisinfo@ucdavis.edu
> Web site: som.ucdavis.edu

University of California - Irvine*
> School of Medicine, Office of Admissions, Berk Hall
> Irvine, California 92697-4089
> Phone: (800) 824-5388
> E-mail: medadmit@uci.edu
> Web site: www.ucihs.uci.edu/com

University of California - Los Angeles*
> David Geffen School of Medicine
> Office of Admissions, Box 957035
> Los Angeles, California 90095-7035
> Phone: (310) 825-6081
> E-mail: somadmiss@mednet.ucla.edu
> Web site: dgsom.healthsciences.ucla.edu/admissions

University of California - San Diego*
School of Medicine, Office of Admissions
0621 Medical Teaching Facility, 9500 Gilman Drive
La Jolla, California 92093-0621
Phone: (858) 534-3880
E-mail: somadmissions@ucsd.edu
Web site: meded.ucsd.edu/admissions/

University of California - San Francisco*
School of Medicine
Office of Admissions, C-200, Box 0408
San Francisco, California 94143
Phone: (415) 476-4044
E-mail: admissions@medsch.ucsf.edu
Web site: medschool.ucsf.edu

University of Southern California*
Keck School of Medicine, Office of Admissions
1975 Zonal Avenue, KAM 100-C
Los Angeles, California 90089-9021
Phone: (323) 442-2552
E-mail: medadmit@usc.edu
Web site: www.usc.edu/schools/medicine

COLORADO

University of Colorado Health Sciences Center - Denver*
School of Medicine
Medical School Admissions Office
4200 East 9th Avenue, C-290
Denver, Colorado 80262
Phone: (303) 315-7361
E-mail: SOMadmin@uchsc.edu
Web site: www.uchsc.edu/sm/sm/

CONNECTICUT

University of Connecticut*
School of Medicine, Student Services Admissions Center
263 Farmington Avenue, Room AG-062
Farmington, Connecticut 06030-3906
Phone: (860) 679-4713
E-mail: fox@nso1.uchc.edu, Sanford@nso1.uchc.edu
Web site: medicine.uchc.edu

Yale University*
School of Medicine, Office of Admissions
Edward S. Harkness Hall, 367 Cedar Street
New Haven, Connecticut 06510

Phone: (203) 785-2696
E-mail: medical.admissions@yale.edu
Web site: info.med.yale.edu/ysm/

The George Washington University*
        School of Medicine and Health Sciences
        Office of Medical School Admissions
        2300 I Street, NW, Walter G. Ross Hall Room 716
        Washington, DC 20037
        Phone: (202) 994-3506
        E-mail: medadmit@gwu.edu
        Web site: www.gwumc.edu/smhs

Georgetown University*
        School of Medicine, Office of Admissions, Box 571421
        Washington, DC 20057-1421
        Phone: (202) 687-1154
        E-mail: medicaladmissions@georgetown.edu
        Web site: som.georgetown.edu

Howard University*
        College of Medicine, Office of Admissions, 520 W Street, NW
        Washington, DC 20059
        Phone: (202) 806-6270
        E-mail: shumphrey@howard.edu
        Web site: www.med.howard.edu

Florida State University*
        College of Medicine
        Admissions Office, 1115 West Call Street
        Tallahassee, Florida 32306-4300
        Phone: (850) 644-7904
        E-mail: medadmissions@med.fsu.edu
        Web site: www.med.fsu.edu

University of Florida*
        College of Medicine, Office of Admissions
        Box 100216, Health Science Center
        Gainesville, Florida 32610-0216
        Phone: (352) 392-4569
        E-mail: robyn@dean.med.ufl.edu
        Web site: www.med.ufl.edu/oea/admiss/

University of Miami*
>Leonard M. Miller School of Medicine
>Office of Admissions, P.O. Box 016159
>Miami, Florida 33101
>Phone: (305) 243-6791
>E-mail: med.admissions@miami.edu
>Web site: www.med.miami.edu

University of South Florida*
>College of Medicine, Office of Admissions / MDC-3
>12901 Bruce B. Downs Boulevard
>Tampa, Florida 33612-4799
>Phone: (813) 974-2229
>E-mail: md-admissions@lyris.hsc.usf.edu
>Web site: www.hsc.usf.edu

GEORGIA

Emory University*
>School of Medicine, Office of Admissions
>Woodruff Health Science Center Administration Building
>1440 Clifton Road, Suite 115
>Atlanta, Georgia 30322-4510
>Phone: (404) 727-5660
>E-mail: medadmiss@emory.edu
>Web site: www.med.emory.edu

Medical College of Georgia*
>School of Medicine, Office of Admissions
>AA-2040, 1120 15th Street
>Augusta, Georgia 30912-4760
>Phone: (706) 721-3186
>E-mail: sclmed.stdadmin@mcg.edu
>Web site: www.mcg.edu

Mercer University*
>School of Medicine, Office of Admissions and Student Affairs
>1550 College Street
>Macon, Georgia 31207-0001
>Phone: (478) 301-2542
>E-mail: Putnam_mc@mercer.edu
>Web site: medicine.mercer.edu

Morehouse School of Medicine*
>School of Medicine, Office of Admissions and Student Affairs
>720 Westview Drive, S.W.
>Atlanta, Georgia 30310-1495

Phone: (404) 752-1650
E-mail: mdadmissions@msm.edu
Web site: www.msm.edu

University of Hawaii*
        John A. Burns School of Medicine
        Office of Student Affairs and Admissions
        Medical Education Building, 651 Ilalo Street
        Honolulu, Hawaii 96813-5534
        Phone: (808) 692-1000
        E-mail: sizutsu@hawaii.edu
        Web site: jabsom.hawaii.edu

Rosalind Franklin University of Medicine and Science*
        Chicago School of Medicine
        Office of Admissions, 3333 Green Bay Road
        North Chicago, Illinois 60064
        Phone: (847) 578-3204
        E-mail: cms.admissions@rosalindfranklin.edu
        Web site: www.rosalindfranklin.edu/cms

Loyola University of Chicago*
        Stritch School of Medicine
        Admissions Office, 2160 South First Avenue
        Maywood, Illinois 60153
        Phone: (708) 216-3229
        E-mail: not available
        Web site: www.meddean.luc.edu

Northwestern University*
        The Feinberg School of Medicine, Office of Admissions
        303 East Chicago Avenue, Morton Building I-606
        Chicago, Illinois 60611-3008
        Phone: (312) 503-8206
        E-mail: med-admissions@northwestern.edu
        Web site: www.medschool.northwestern.edu

Rush University*
        Rush Medical College, Office of Admissions
        Suite 524-H, 600 South Paulina Street
        Chicago, Illinois 60612-3832
        Phone: (312) 942-6913
        E-mail: RMC_Admissions@rush.edu
        Web site: www.rushu.rush.edu/medcol

Southern Illinois University*
 School of Medicine, Office of Student Affairs, P.O. Box 19624
 Springfield, Illinois 62794-9624
 Phone: (217) 545-6013
 E-mail: admissions@siumed.edu
 Web site: www.siumed.edu

University of Chicago*
 The Pritzker School of Medicine
 Office of Admissions, 924 East 57th Street, Suite 104
 Chicago, Illinois 60637-5415
 Phone: (773) 702-1939
 E-mail: pritzkeradmissions@bsd.uchicago.edu
 Web site: pritzker.bsd.uchicago.edu/

University of Illinois*
 College of Medicine, Office of Admissions
 808 South Wood Street, MC-783, Room 165 CME
 Chicago, Illinois 60612-7302
 Phone: (312) 996-5635
 E-mail: medadmit@uic.edu
 Web site: www.medicine.uic.edu

INDIANA

Indiana University*
 School of Medicine, Medical School Admissions Office
 1120 South Drive, Fesler Hall 213
 Indianapolis, Indiana 46202-5113
 Phone: (317) 274-3772
 E-mail: inmedadm@iupui.edu
 Web site: www.medicine.iu.edu

IOWA

University of Iowa*
 Roy J. & Lucille A. Carver College of Medicine
 Admissions, 100 Medicine Administration Building
 Iowa City, Iowa 52242-1101
 Phone: (319) 335-8052
 E-mail: medical-admissions@uiowa.edu
 Web site: www.medicine.uiowa.edu

KANSAS

University of Kansas*
 School of Medicine, Office of Admissions
 Mail Stop 1049, 3901 Rainbow Boulevard
 Kansas City, Kansas 66160
 Phone: (913) 588-5245
 E-mail: premedinfo@kumc.edu
 Web site: www.kumc.edu/som/

KENTUCKY

University of Kentucky*
College of Medicine, Office of Admissions
MN-118 Chandler Medical Center
Lexington, Kentucky 40536-0298
Phone: (859) 323-6161
E-mail: kymedap@uky.edu
Web site: www.mc.uky.edu/medicine

University of Louisville*
School of Medicine, Office of Admissions
Abell Administration Center, 323 East Chestnut Street
Louisville, Kentucky 40202-3866
Phone: (502) 852-5193
E-mail: medadm@louisville.edu
Web site: www.louisville.edu/medschool

LOUISIANA

Louisiana State University - New Orleans*
School of Medicine, Student Admissions
1901 Perdido Street, Box P3-4
New Orleans, Louisiana 70112-1393
Phone: (504) 568-6262
E-mail: ms-admissions@lsuhsc.edu
Web site: www.medschool.lsuhsc.edu

Louisiana State University Health Sciences Center - Shreveport*
School of Medicine, Student Admissions, P.O. Box 33932
Shreveport, Louisiana 71130-3932
Phone: (318) 675-5190
E-mail: shvadm@lsuhsc.edu
Web site: www.sh.lsuhsc.edu/index.html

Tulane University*
School of Medicine, Office of Admissions and Student Affairs
1430 Tulane Avenue, SL67
New Orleans, Louisiana 70112-2699
Phone: (504) 988-5462
E-mail: medsch@tulane.edu
Web site: www.som.tulane.edu

MARYLAND

The Johns Hopkins University*
School of Medicine, Office of Admissions
733 North Broadway, Suite G-49
Baltimore, Maryland 21205-2196
Phone: (410) 955-3182
E-mail: somadmiss@jhmi.edu
Web site: www.hopkinsmedicine.org/som

Uniformed Services University of the Health Sciences*
    F. Edward Hebert School of Medicine
    Office of Admissions, Room A-1041, 301 Jones Bridge Road
    Bethesda, Maryland 20814-4799
    Phone: (301) 295-3101
    E-mail: admissions@mxa.usuhs.mil
    Web site: www.usuhs.mil

University of Maryland*
    School of Medicine
    Health Sciences Facility I, Office of Admissions
    685 West Baltimore Street, Suite 190
    Baltimore, Maryland 21201-1559
    Phone: (410) 706-7478
    E-mail: admissions@som.umaryland.edu
    Web site: www.medschool.umaryland.edu

MASSACHUSETTS

Boston University*
    School of Medicine, Office of Admissions, L-124
    715 Albany Street
    Boston, Massachusetts 02118
    Phone: (617) 638-4630
    E-mail: medadms@bu.edu
    Web site: www.bumc.bu.edu/busm/

Harvard Medical School*
    Office of the Committee on Admissions, 25 Shattuck Street
    Boston, Massachusetts 02115-6092
    Phone: (617) 432-1550
    E-mail: admissions_office@hms.harvard.edu
    Web site: hms.harvard.edu

Tufts University*
    School of Medicine, Office of Admissions
    136 Harrison Avenue
    Boston, Massachusetts 02111
    Phone: (617) 636-6571
    E-mail: med-admissions@tufts.edu
    Web site: www.tufts.edu/med

University of Massachusetts*
    School of Medicine, Office of Admissions
    55 Lake Avenue, North, Room S1-112
    Worcester, Massachusetts 01655
    Phone: (508) 856-2323
    E-mail: admissions@umassmed.edu
    Web site: www.umassmed.edu/education

MICHIGAN

Michigan State University*
    College of Human Medicine, Office of Admissions
    A-239 Life Sciences Building
    East Lansing, Michigan 48824-1317
    Phone: (517) 353-9620
    E-mail: MDadmissions@msu.edu
    Web site: humanmedicine.msu.edu/

University of Michigan*
    Medical School, Office of Admissions
    4303 Medical Science Building I, 1310 Catherine Road
    Ann Arbor, Michigan 48109-0624
    Phone: (734) 764-6317
    E-mail: umichmedadmiss@umich.edu
    Web site: www.med.umich.edu/medschool

Wayne State University*
    School of Medicine, Office of Admissions
    540 East Canfield Street, 1310 Scott Hall
    Detroit, Michigan 48201
    Phone: (313) 577-1466
    E-mail: admissions@med.wayne.edu
    Web site: www.med.wayne.edu

MINNESOTA

Mayo Medical School*
    200 First Street, SW
    Rochester, Minnesota 55905
    Phone: (507) 284-3671
    E-mail: MedSchoolAdmissions@mayo.edu
    Web site: www.mayo.edu/mms

University of Minnesota*
    Medical School, Office of Admissions
    Mayo Mail Code # 293, 420 Delaware Street SE
    Minneapolis, Minnesota 55455
    Phone: (612) 625-7977
    E-mail: meded@umn.edu
    Web site: www.med.umn.edu/

MISSISSIPPI

The University of Mississippi Medical Center*
    School of Medicine, Office of Admissions
    2500 North State Street
    Jackson, Mississippi 39216-4505
    Phone: (601) 984-5010
    E-mail: AdmitMD@som.umsmed.edu
    Web site: som.umc.edu

Saint Louis University*
  School of Medicine, Office of Admissions
  1402 South Grand Boulevard. M226
  St. Louis, Missouri 63104
  Phone: (314) 977-9870
  E-mail: slumd@slu.edu
  Web site: medschool.slu.edu

University of Missouri – Columbia*
  School of Medicine
  Admissions, Recruitment, and Records Coordinator
  Office of Medical Education
  MA215 Medical Science Building, One Hospital Drive
  Columbia, Missouri 65212
  Phone: (573) 882-9219
  E-mail: nolkej@health.missouri.edu
  Web site: www.muhealth.org/~medicine

University of Missouri - Kansas City (UMKC):   **No AMCAS**
  School of Medicine, Council on Selection, 2411 Holmes Road
  Kansas City, Missouri 64108-2792
  Phone: (816) 235-1870
  E-mail: umkcmedweb@umkc.edu
  Web site: www.umkc.edu/medicine

The UMKC School of Medicine is designed primarily for high school graduates. Students will earn their baccalaureate and M.D. degrees concurrently during a six-year program.

Washington University in St. Louis*
  School of Medicine, Office of Admissions
  660 South Euclid Avenue, Campus Box 8107
  St. Louis, Missouri 63110-1093
  Phone: (314) 362-6858
  E-mail: wumscoa@wustl.edu
  Web site: www.medicine.wustl.edu

Creighton University*
  School of Medicine, Office of Medical Admissions
  Criss III, Room 574, 2500 California Plaza
  Omaha, Nebraska 68178

Phone: (402) 280-2799
E-mail: medschadm@creighton.edu
Web site: medicine.creighton.edu

University of Nebraska*
       College of Medicine, Office of Admissions and Students
       986585 Nebraska Medical Center
       Omaha, Nebraska 68198-6585
       Phone: (402) 559-2259
       E-mail: grrogers@unmc.edu
       Web site: www.unmc.edu/uncom

NEVADA

University of Nevada*
       School of Medicine
       Office of Admissions and Student Affairs, Mail Stop 357
       Reno, Nevada 89557-0129
       Phone: (775) 784-6063
       E-mail: asa@med.unr.edu
       Web site: www.unr.edu/med

NEW HAMPSHIRE

Dartmouth Medical School*
       Office of Admissions, 3 Rope Ferry Road
       Hanover, New Hampshire 03755-1404
       Phone: (603) 650-1505
       E-mail: dms.admissions@dartmouth.edu
       Web site: www.dms.dartmouth.edu

NEW JERSEY

University of Medicine and Dentistry of New Jersey*
       Office of Admissions, 185 South Orange Avenue
       Room C-653, P.O. Box 1709
       Newark, New Jersey 07103
       Phone: (973) 972-4631
       E-mail: njmsadmiss@umdnj.edu
       Web site: njms.umdnj.edu

University of Medicine and Dentistry of New Jersey – Robert
Wood Johnson Medical School*
       Office of Admissions, 675 Hoes Lane
       Piscataway, New Jersey 08854-5635
       Phone: (732) 235-4576
       E-mail: rwjapadm@umdnj.edu
       Web site: rwjms.umdnj.edu

NEW MEXICO

University of New Mexico*
School of Medicine, Office of Admissions, MSC084690
Basic Medical Sciences Building, Room 106
Albuquerque, New Mexico 87131-0001
Phone: (505) 272-4766
E-mail: somadmissions@salud.unm.edu
Web site: hsc.unm.edu/som

NEW YORK

Albany Medical College*
Admissions Office, Mail Code 3, 47 New Scotland Avenue
Albany, New York 12208-3479
Phone: (518) 262-5521
E-mail: admissions@mail.amc.edu
Web site: www.amc.edu/Academic/Aboutcollege/

Albert Einstein of Yeshiva University*
Albert Einstein College of Medicine
Office of Admissions, Belfer Building, Room 211
1300 Morris Park Avenue
Bronx, New York 10461
Phone: (718) 430-2106
E-mail: admissions@aecom.yu.edu
Web site: www.aecom.yu.edu

Columbia University*
College of Physicians and Surgeons, Admissions Office
630 West 168th Street, Box 41, Room 1-416
New York, New York 10032
Phone: (212) 305-3595
E-mail: psadmissions@columbia.edu
Web site: cumc.columbia.edu/dept/ps

Weill Cornell Medical College*
Weill Medical College, Office of Admissions
445 East 69th Street, Room 104
New York, New York 10021
Phone: (212) 746-1067
E-mail: cumc-admissions@med.cornell.edu
Web site: www.med.cornell.edu

Mount Sinai School of Medicine*
School of Medicine, Office of Admissions
Annenberg Building, Room 5-04
One Gustave L. Levy Place – Box 1002
New York, New York 10029-6574

Phone: (212) 241-6696
E-mail: admissions@mssm.edu
Web site: www.mssm.edu

New York Medical College*
    Office of Admissions, Administration Building, Room 147
    Sunshine Cottage Road
    Valhalla, New York 10595
    Phone: (914) 594-4507
    E-mail: mdadmit@nymc.edu
    Web site: www.nymc.edu

New York University*
    School of Medicine, Office of Admissions, 550 First Avenue
    New York, New York 10016
    Phone: (212) 263-5290
    E-mail: admissions@med.nyu.edu
    Web site: www.med.nyu.edu

State University of New York University at Buffalo*
    School of Medicine and Biomedical Sciences
    Office of Medical Admissions
    131 Biomedical Education Building
    Buffalo, New York 14214-3013
    Phone: (716) 829-3466
    E-mail: jjrosso@buffalo.edu
    Web site: www.smbs.buffalo.edu

State University of New York Downstate Medical Center*
    College of Medicine, Admissions Office
    450 Clarkson Avenue, Box 60
    Brooklyn, New York 11203-2098
    Phone: (718) 270-2446
    E-mail: admissions@downstate.edu
    Web site: www.downstate.edu

State University of New York Upstate Medical University*
    College of Medicine, Admissions Office
    1215 Weiskotten Hall, 766 Irving Avenue
    Syracuse, New York 13210
    Phone: (315) 464-4570
    E-mail: admiss@upstate.edu
    Web site: www.upstate.edu/com

State University of New York Stony Brook University Medical Center*
School of Medicine, Office of Admissions
Health Sciences Level 4
Stony Brook, New York 11794-8434
Phone: (631) 444-2113
E-mail: somadmissions@stonybrook.edu
Web site: www.hsc.sunysb.edu/som

University of Rochester*
School of Medicine, Office of Admissions
601 Elmwood Avenue, Box 601A
Rochester, New York 14642
Phone: (585) 275-4539
E-mail: mdadmish@urmc.rochester.edu
Web site: www.urmc.rochester.edu/SMD

NORTH CAROLINA

East Carolina University*
The Brody School of Medicine
600 Moye Boulevard, Office of Admissions
Greenville, North Carolina 27834
Phone: (252) 744-2202
E-mail: somadmissions@mail.ecu.edu
Web site: www.ecu.edu/med

Duke University*
School of Medicine, Office of Admissions
Duke University Medical Center, Box 3710
Durham, North Carolina 27710
Phone: (919) 684-2985
E-mail: medadm@mc.duke.edu
Web site: dukemed.duke.edu

University of North Carolina - Chapel Hill*
School of Medicine, Office of Admissions
CB #9500 1001 Bondurant Hall, First Floor
Chapel Hill, North Carolina 27599-9500
Phone: (919) 962-8331
E-mail: Admis_UNC_SOM@listserv.med.unc.edu
Web site: www.med.unc.edu

Wake Forest University*
School of Medicine, Office of Medical School Admissions
Medical Center Boulevard
Winston-Salem, North Carolina 27157-1090

```
Phone:      (336) 716-4264
E-mail:     medadmit@wfubmc.edu
Web site:   www.wfubmc.edu/school
```

NORTH DAKOTA

University of North Dakota
    School of Medicine and Health Sciences
    Committee on Admissions
    501 North Columbia Road, STOP 9037
    Grand Forks, North Dakota 58202-9037
```
Phone:      (701) 777-4221
E-mail:     jdheit@medicine.nodak.edu
Web site:   www.med.und.nodak.edu
```

OHIO

Case Western Reserve University*
    School of Medicine, Office of Admissions, T308
    2109 Adelbert Road
    Cleveland, Ohio 44106-4920
```
Phone:      (216) 368-3450
E-mail:     casemed-admissions@case.edu
Web site:   casemed.case.edu
```

Medical University of Ohio - Toledo*
    College of Medicine, Admissions Office
    3045 Arlington Avenue
    Toledo, Ohio 43614
```
Phone:      (419) 383-4229
E-mail:     admissions@meduohio.edu
Web site:   www.meduohio.edu
```

Northeastern Ohio Universities*
    College of Medicine, Office of Admissions
    4209 State Route 44, P.O. Box 95
    Rootstown, Ohio 44272-0095
```
Phone:      (330) 325-6270
E-mail:     admission@neoucom.edu
Web site:   www.neoucom.edu
```

The Ohio State University*
    College of Medicine, Admissions Committee
    155D Meiling Hall, 370 West 9th Avenue
    Columbus, Ohio 43210-1238
```
Phone:      (614) 292-7137
E-mail:     medicine@osu.edu
Web site:   medicine.osu.edu
```

University of Cincinnati*
 College of Medicine, Office of Admissions
 231 Albert Sabin Way, Room E251, MSB
 Cincinnati, Ohio 45267-0552
 Phone: (513) 558-7314
 E-mail: comadmis@ucmail.uc.edu
 Web site: www.med.uc.edu

Wright State University*
 Boonshoft School of Medicine
 Office of Student Affairs and Admissions, P.O. Box 1751
 Dayton, Ohio 45401-1751
 Phone: (937) 775-2936
 E-mail: som_saa@wright.edu
 Web site: www.med.wright.edu

OKLAHOMA

University of Oklahoma*
 College of Medicine, Office of Admissions
 P.O. Box 26901, BMSB 357
 Oklahoma City, Oklahoma 73190
 Phone: (405) 271-2331
 E-mail: adminmed@ouhsc.edu
 Web site: www.medicine.ouhsc.edu

OREGON

Oregon Health and Science University*
 School of Medicine, Office of Admissions
 3181 SW Sam Jackson Park Road
 Portland, Oregon 97239
 Phone: (503) 494-2998
 E-mail: not available
 Web site: www.ohsu.edu/som

PENNSYLVANIA

Drexel University*
 College of Medicine, Office of Admissions, 2900 Queen Lane
 Philadelphia, Pennsylvania 19129
 Phone: (215) 991-8202
 E-mail: medadmis@drexel.edu
 Web site: www.drexelmed.edu

Thomas Jefferson University*
 Jefferson Medical College, Admissions Office
 1015 Walnut Street, Suite 110
 Philadelphia, Pennsylvania 19107-5099
 Phone: (215) 955-6983
 E-mail: jmc.admissions@jefferson.edu
 Web site: www.jefferson.edu/jmc

The Pennsylvania State University*
    College of Medicine, Office of Medical Student Affairs, H060
    500 University Drive, P.O. Box 850
    Hershey, Pennsylvania 17033
    Phone: (717) 531-8755
    E-mail: studentadmissions@hmc.psu.edu
    Web site: www.hmc.psu.edu/md

Temple University*
    School of Medicine, Office of Admissions
    3340 N. Broad Street, SFC, Suite 305
    Philadelphia, Pennsylvania 19140
    Phone: (215) 707-3656
    E-mail: medadmissions@temple.edu
    Web site: www.temple.edu/medicine

University of Pennsylvania*
    School of Medicine, Office of Admissions
    Suite 100, Edward J. Stemmler Hall, 3450 Hamilton Walk
    Philadelphia, Pennsylvania 19104-6056
    Phone: (215) 898-8001
    E-mail: admiss@mail.med.upenn.edu
    Web site: www.med.upenn.edu

University of Pittsburgh*
    School of Medicine, Office of Admissions and Financial Aid
    518 Scaife Hall, 3550 Terrace Street
    Pittsburgh, Pennsylvania 15261
    Phone: (412) 648-9891
    E-mail: admissions@medschool.pitt.edu
    Web site: www.medschool.pitt.edu

PUERTO RICO

Ponce School of Medicine*
    Admissions Office, P.O. Box 7004
    Ponce, Puerto Rico 00732
    Phone: (787) 840-2575
    E-mail: admissions@psm.edu
    Web site: www.psm.edu

Universidad Central del Caribe*
    School of Medicine, Office of Admissions, P.O. Box 60-327
    Bayamon, Puerto Rico 00960-6032
    Phone: (787) 798-3001
    E-mail: icordero@uccaribe.edu
    Web site: www.uccaribe.edu

University of Puerto Rico*
> School of Medicine, Central Admissions Office
> Medical Sciences Campus, P.O. Box 365067
> San Juan, Puerto Rico 00936-5067
> Phone: (787) 758-2525
> E-mail: marrivera@rcm.upr.edu
> Web site: medweb.rcm.upr.edu

RHODE ISLAND

Brown University*
> School of Medicine, Office of Admissions and Financial Aid
> 97 Waterman Street, Box G-A213
> Providence, Rhode Island 02912-9706
> Phone: (401) 863-2149
> E-mail: MedSchool_Admissions@brown.edu
> Web site: bms.brown.edu

SOUTH CAROLINA

Medical University of South Carolina*
> College of Medicine, Dean's Office
> 96 Jonathan Lucas Street, Suite 601, P.O. Box 250617
> Charleston, South Carolina 29425
> Phone: (843) 792-2055
> E-mail: taylorwl@musc.edu
> Web site: www.musc.edu

University of South Carolina*
> School of Medicine, Office of Admissions
> Columbia, South Carolina 29208
> Phone: (803) 733-3325
> E-mail: jeanette@gw.med.sc.edu
> Web site: www.med.sc.edu

SOUTH DAKOTA

University of South Dakota*
> Sanford School of Medicine
> Medical School Admissions, 414 East Clark Street
> Vermillion, South Dakota 57069-2390
> Phone: (605) 677-5233
> E-mail: usdsmsa@usd.edu
> Web site: www.usd.edu/med/md

TENNESSEE

East Tennessee State University*
> James H. Quillen College of Medicine
> Office of Admissions, P.O. Box 70580
> Johnson City, Tennessee 37614-1708
> Phone: (423) 439-2033
> E-mail: sacom@etsu.edu
> Web site: com.etsu.edu

Meharry Medical College*
Office of Admissions, 1005 Dr. D. B. Todd, Jr. Boulevard
Nashville, Tennessee 37208-3599
Phone: (615) 327-6223
E-mail: admissions@mmc.edu
Web site: www.mmc.edu

University of Tennessee Health Science Center*
College of Medicine, Admissions Office
Medical Center Plaza, 910 Madison Avenue, Suite 500
Memphis, Tennessee 38163
Phone: (901) 448-5559
E-mail: nstrother@utmem.edu
Web site: www.utmem.edu/Medicine

Vanderbilt University*
School of Medicine, Office of Admissions, 215 Light Hall
Nashville, Tennessee 37232-0685
Phone: (615) 322-2145
E-mail: pat.sagen@vanderbilt.edu
Web site: www.mc.vanderbilt.edu/medschool

TEXAS

Baylor College of Medicine*
Office of Admissions, One Baylor Plaza
Room N104, MS-BCM 110
Houston, Texas 77030
Phone: (713) 798-4842
E-mail: admissions@bcm.edu
Web site: www.bcm.edu

Students applying to any of the following six allopathic
medical schools must apply through TMDSAS.

Texas A&M University System Health Science Center
College of Medicine, Office of Student Affairs and Admissions
159 Reynolds Medical Building
College Station, Texas 77843-1114
Phone: (979) 845-7743
E-mail: admissions@medicine.tamhsc.edu
Web site: www.medicine.tamhsc.edu

Texas Tech. University Health Sciences Center
    School of Medicine, Office of Admissions
    Room 2B116, 3601 4th Street
    Lubbock, Texas 79430
    Phone: (806) 743-2297
    E-mail: somadm@ttuhsc.edu
    Web site: www.ttuhsc.edu

University of Texas Medical Branch at Galveston
    Office of Admissions, 301 University Boulevard
    Galveston, Texas 77555-1317
    Phone: (409) 772-6958
    E-mail: tsilva@utmb.edu
    Web site: www.som.utmb.edu

University of Texas at Houston
    Medical School, Office of Admissions, Room G.420
    6431 Fannin Street, MSB G.420
    Houston, Texas 77030
    Phone: (713) 500-5116
    E-mail: msadmissions@uth.tmc.edu
    Web site: www.med.uth.tmc.edu

University of Texas Health Science Center at San Antonio
    School of Medicine, Office of Admissions
    7703 Floyd Curl Drive
    San Antonio, Texas 78229-3900
    Phone: (210) 567-6080
    E-mail: MedAdmissions@uthscsa.edu
    Web site: som.uthscsa.edu

University of Texas Southwestern Medical Center at Dallas
    Admissions Office, 5323 Harry Hines Boulevard
    Dallas, Texas 75390-9162
    Phone: (214) 648-5617
    E-mail: admissions@utsouthwestern.edu
    Web site: www.utsouthwestern.edu

UTAH

University of Utah*
    School of Medicine, Office of Admissions
    30 North 1900 East, Room 1C029
    Salt Lake City, Utah 84132-2101
    Phone: (801) 581-7498
    E-mail: deans.admissions@hsc.utah.edu
    Web site: uuhsc.utah.edu/som

University of Vermont*
    College of Medicine, Office of Admissions
    E-215 Given Building, 89 Beaumont Avenue
    Burlington, Vermont 05405
    Phone: (802) 656-2154
    E-mail: MedAdmissions@uvm.edu
    Web site: www.med.uvm.edu

Eastern Virginia Medical School*
    Office of Admissions, 700 West Olney Road
    Norfolk, Virginia 23507-1607
    Phone: (757) 446-5812
    E-mail: nanezkf@evms.edu
    Web site: www.evms.edu

University of Virginia Health System*
    School of Medicine, Admissions Office, P.O. Box 800725
    Charlottesville, Virginia 22908
    Phone: (434) 924-5571
    E-mail: medsch-adm@virginia.edu
    Web site: www.hsc.virginia.edu

Virginia Commonwealth University*
    School of Medicine, Office of Admissions
    1101 East Marshall Street, P.O. Box 980565
    Richmond, Virginia 23298-0565
    Phone: (804) 828-9629
    E-mail: somadm@vcu.edu
    Web site: www.medschool.vcu.edu

University of Washington*
    School of Medicine, Office of Admissions
    A-300 Health Sciences Building, Box 356340
    Seattle, Washington 98195-6340
    Phone: (206) 543-7212
    E-mail: askuwsom@u.washington.edu
    Web site: www.uwmedicine.org

Marshall University*
    Joan C. Edwards School of Medicine
    Admissions Office, 1600 Medical Center Drive
    Huntington, West Virginia 25701-3655
    Phone: (800) 544-8514
    E-mail: warren@marshall.edu
    Web site: musom.marshall.edu

West Virginia University*
    School of Medicine, Office of Student Services
    Byrd Health Sciences Center, P.O. Box 9111
    Morgantown, West Virginia 26506
    Phone: (304) 293-1439
    E-mail: medadmissions@hsc.wvu.edu
    Web site: www.hsc.wvu.edu/som

WISCONSIN

Medical College of Wisconsin*
    Office of Admissions, 8701 Watertown Plank Road
    Milwaukee, Wisconsin 53226
    Phone: (414) 456-8246
    E-mail: medschool@mcw.edu
    Web site: www.mcw.edu

University of Wisconsin*
    School of Medicine, Admissions Committee
    2130 Health Sciences Learning Center
    750 Highland Avenue
    Madison, Wisconsin 53705-2221
    Phone: (608) 263-4925
    E-mail: medadmissions@wisc.edu
    Web site: www.med.wisc.edu